AN ELEMENTARY TEXTBOOK OF AYURVEDA

AN ELEMENTARY TEXTBOOK OF AYURVEDA:

MEDICINE WITH A SIX THOUSAND YEAR OLD TRADITION

Frank John Ninivaggi, M.D.

Psychosocial Press
Madison Connecticut

Library of Congress Cataloging-in-Publication Data

Ninivaggi, Frank John.
An elementary textbook of Ayurveda : medicine with a six thousand year old tradition /
Frank John Ninivaggi.
p. cm.
Includes bibliographical references.
ISBN 1-887841-33-4
1. Medicine, Ayurvedic. I. Title.

R605.N49 2001
615.5'3–dc21

00-051725

Manufactured in the United States of America

CONTENTS

Chapter 7. Health and the Disease Process. II

Chapter 8. Nutrition and Diet in Ayurveda

INTRODUCTION

Ayurveda, life wisdom, is an ancient yet living discipline. Its theories and methods combine the ordinary with the extraordinary. Adherents of Ayurveda believe that its origins extend back at least 6,000 years. There is some inferential evidence to support this contention. Others say that a 3,000-year-old legacy is clearly verifiable. It would not be an understatement to regard Ayurveda as a world-class system of health and well-being. If this is true, one then wonders why its recognition as such in the West has been so delayed. Ayurveda, an ancient Sanskrit word, derives from the traditions of the ancient Indian *rishis* (sages) and denotes the enlightened knowledge of all aspects of optimal, healthy, everyday living, and longevity. Its adherents consider it a "fortress of wisdom."

A factor responsible for the slow recognition of Ayurvedic wisdom in the West may be the intentional ambiguity in form and content that has characterized its prehistory, history, and development. Its practical relevance for the Westerner may also be unclear. Eastern ideas have always been clothed in fluid boundaries and their content may have appeared amorphous, intangible, impractical, and speculative, if not fanciful to Western thinkers. Among Ayurveda's primary values are the concepts of *Sattva* and of *Dharma*.

The Sanskrit word *sattva* refers to the ongoing attainment of ever-greater degrees of purity, harmony, balance, and goodness in one's life. For Hindus, the Sanskrit word *dharma,* an equally broad notion, refers to an individual's recognition of inherent lawfulness in the universe, assuming personal responsibility, and taking charge of one's own life in the world. In the Buddhist tradition, which emerged out of Hinduism in the sixth century B.C., the term *dharma* refers to the entire body of teachings, the corpus of enlightened life wisdom, ascribed to the Buddha. In fact, one of the great luminaries of Ayurveda, Nagarjuna (c. second century A.D.), was both an Ayurvedic physician and a Buddhist priest. The breadth of his wisdom not only enriched the Ayurvedic Materia Media in a pragmatic way with the introduction of iatrochemistry (mineral-based medicine), but advanced the scope of Buddhism with contributions having profound philosophical and psychological significance. The inestimable significance and living historicity of Nagarjuna's contributions attest to his continuing to be a creative Ayurvedic presence, a golden thread stretching back two millennia.

The range of Ayurvedic thinking covers thousands of years of ideas, practical experience, and theory building. It is hoped that this *Elementary Textbook of Ayurveda* will not inadvertently oversimplify the profound depth of this ancient medical system but, instead, present its basic elements in a scholarly, yet reverent and compassionate, fashion to the serious reader. Ayurveda truly is more than merely Indian medical science. It is, in fact, a universally applicable way of life that addresses all aspects of living both in health and in disease. Practitioners of this art frequently refer to it as being proven over time. Ongoing experience, however, does and will continue to suggest, short of scientific proof, degrees of validity in the Ayurvedic worldview.

The history and development of Indian culture is famous for introducing and entertaining a multiplicity of widely divergent worldviews. Disputes abound concerning the nature and meaning of the individual's place in the world, of personal identity, of pluralism versus monism, and of a personal Deity or a more transcendent Absolute. For Ayurveda, reality consists of a universe of animate and inanimate beings, all of which are grounded in a primordial matrix of immaterial consciousness. The Sanskrit term that covers the entire range of all that exists is *Brahman*, the one absolute reality. The ancient Vedic scriptures repeatedly stressed the point that ontologically, "everything is *Brahman*" (*sarvam khalvidam Brahma*) and "all is *Brahman*" (*kham*

Brahm). This view especially pertained to man; his essence was seen to be identical with *Brahman* (*Tat Tvam Asi*). This unifying monism is central to Ayurveda. Moreover, in like fashion to most other philosophical, religious, spiritual, humanistic, and healing ideologies, Ayurveda centers its attention almost entirely on man and the meaningfulness of his existence in the world. Man's place in the universe is an essential theme. The role of man on earth, in society, within the family, interpersonally, and with himself, per se, is viewed as a proper and necessary concern, and not as an archaic, anthropomorphic, and fanciful self-indulgence.

The Ayurvedic system delineates a way of life for human beings which enables them to address all aspects of self-development. Self-inquiry, self-realization, and self-actualization are central themes. A strong emphasis is put on the individual's mandated responsibility (*dharma*) for himself; he must actively take charge of his own well-being. The interpersonal and social aspect of this resides in the belief that when one fulfills one's own *dharma* (personal and social duties), one also benefits the immediate and extended social group. In addition, Ayurveda sees the surrounding natural world (animals, minerals, seasons, etc.) as being sacred, and uses aspects of it in an ecologically respectful manner to further the welfare of both man and nature. This conception is mirrored in the Ayurvedic theory of the five Elements, a delineated matrix of five material principles within nature that make up all animate and inanimate bodies.

Personal change and transformation are among Ayurveda's central concerns. This covers change in both the psychological and the physical domains. Both aspects are pressing since they repeatedly present the individual with an apparently rebellious and persistent tendency to go awry, produce malaise, and then spark an impulse toward correction. Man's will, his conative or volitional faculty, is preeminent in implementing this action. All change, in fact, is considered self-change. This idea has two levels of meaning: (1) the abstract cognitive recognition of personal disharmony along with the experience of the impulse to change; and (2) an individual's integrated efforts that result in the material occurrence of actual, concrete change. Some comparisons between Ayurveda and Western medicine may be useful to demonstrate some similarities and differences since issues of disorder and strategies for change are major features of both.

Whereas Western medicine strives for accuracy by using a scientific method and accumulating statistically significant data about health and disease, Ayurveda tends more toward naturalism, that is, an empirical approach closer to nature. This entails a strong, almost exclusive reliance on clinical examination and diagnosis and the absence of any formal laboratory investigations. The linear thinking and logic of Western medicine is highly analytic, categorical, and uses a classification system of discrete disease entities as a basic template to guide the direction of treatment. Most pathological conditions are primarily conceived of as coarse manifestations of actual gross disease processes. By comparison, the central paradigm in Ayurveda is the maintenance of optimal health by daily proactive care. The individual is seen as a comprehensive and integrated biopsychospiritual being who strives for an optimal quality of life by adhering to daily health routines. These include diet, exercise, and psychological work, all of which are continually modified according to seasonal changes. Ayurveda presents a comprehensive way of life that encourages balance in all aspects of living. It proactively treats the subtle, almost imperceptible, trends toward imbalance and their inevitable diatheses toward formal illness using routine prophylactic maintenance. The individual is believed to have an innate capacity for potential self-correction and primary self-healing.

While Western medicine treats discrete disease entities, Ayurveda treats the subtly experienced states of dysphoria and malaise whose insidiously disruptive trends may only later develop into discrete disease entities. The approach of Western medicine, therefore, strives for scientific objectivity and verifiability. Disease and disease states are seen as discrete entities that are superimposed, for the most part, on man. Medical interventions have a relatively more ahistorical and "experience-distant" basis. Ayurveda, on the other hand, is preeminently "experience-near" and holds *pratyaksha,* a direct grasp of the multisensory perceptive understanding of each individual patient, as its foremost diagnostic tool. Disease and illness are understood to be dynamic imbalances that organically emerge out of man's innate constitution as it interacts with the environment over time.

A fair question then becomes: Why consider using Ayurveda when Western medicine has so much to offer? A satisfactory answer is fraught with the complexities that both healing systems intrinsically contain along with the fact of their differing cultural origins. While it may be reasonable to consider that the two health care systems probably may not be capable of immediate theoretical integration at this time, their complementary and adjunctive clinical application seems both reasonable and justifiable. If Ayurveda and Western medicine are used together, pragmatically, their reciprocal interaction could be synergistic and create a greater degree of clinical efficacy. This remains an interesting and open question, and will rest heavily on the skill, ingenuity, and good will of health providers of differing disciplines. Of course, therapeutic results from either or both health systems will naturally result in differential beneficial response rates due to the heterogeneity of patients, diseases, and other intervention variables. Ayurveda, in general, is more geared toward health maintenance rather than disease treatment. It is a system of diet and lifestyle whose aim is to enhance the quality of life by dealing with the subtle trends that might lead to actual disease. It is, therefore, a method for living life in a more fulfilled manner. Quality of life is a high priority.

Lastly, another important consideration would take into account the fact that Ayurveda might not be a useful choice or rather may appear incompatible with the beliefs, values, and motivations of those whose outlooks preclude such naturalistic, spiritual, and consciousness-oriented approaches. Natural and alternative approaches often require intentional and sustained self-discipline, perseverance, and taking an active, personal role in matters of health and overall lifestyle. This self-help approach has not been a part of the traditional Western medical model. In addition, substantive change requires guidance and monitoring from a highly qualified Ayurvedic specialist. This, in itself, may be viewed as arduous since it necessitates commitment over time. Insofar as consciousness and spirituality are inclusive domains within Ayurveda, some may prefer to focus only on the psychological aspects that are an inseparable part of these; others may choose to use only the health practices. These partial approaches are certainly useful and worthwhile. Ayurveda, it will be seen, is not only compatible with virtually all points of view, i.e., health, philosophical, religious, but can even provide one with a more enhanced mindset and state of physical well-being thus affording more receptivity and skill in the particular way of life, e.g., relationship, career, religion, etc., that is already in place.

Ayurveda, like Western medical science, developed subspecialties to address particular medical and health needs. The *Ashtanga Ayurveda* (eight branches or limbs of Ayurveda) are the following:

1. *Kayachikitsa,* Internal Medicine
2. *Shalyatantra,* Surgery
3. *Shalakya Tantra,* Otolaryngology, Ophthalmology
4. *Kaumarabhritya,* Obstetrics, Gynecology, and Pediatrics
5. *Agadatantra,* Toxicology
6. *Bhutavidya,* Psychiatry
7. *Rasayana,* Antiaging and rejuvenation
8. *Vajikarana,* Reproductive and aphrodisiac medicine

This *Elementary Textbook of Ayurveda* will concentrate on the presentation of the theoretical propositions and clinical principles that make up the fundamental Ayurvedic corpus. Sanskrit terms are rendered in a simplified and anglicized manner as is commonly found in nontechnical English transliterations. Particular spellings, formats of phrases, capitalization, etc., have been chosen, to some degree arbitrarily, for the sake of uniformity and to emphasize special significance. A glossary of selected terms, inclusive but not exhaustive, has been provided that contains the basic vocabulary necessary to achieve an adequate grasp of the subject. Not every Sanskrit term used in the text is included in the glossary, either because its significance as a term per se is considered nonessential to an understanding of basic Ayurveda or because it is more properly related to a different specialized field, e.g., Yoga. Following current conventions when presenting Ayurvedic concepts in English-speaking circles, this text attempts to use either the appropriate Sanskrit term or its English meaning in a relatively uniform, though not rigid, fashion. As mentioned earlier, since the breadth of detail in Ayurveda is formidable, only some essential areas will be covered here. These areas and the level of detail presented are, in fact, representative of the substantive matrix of basic Ayurveda. Much important material, of necessity, has been intentionally left out. Two large areas of omission are (1) a detailed account of the herbomineral armamentarium of Ayurvedic Materia Medica; and (2) an exhaustive outline of particular disease states and their remediation. Some popular as well as scholarly publications covering these areas are currently available in English; some of these will be cited in the references. The author has made extensive use of one of Ayurveda's indisputably foundational medical compilations, the *Charaka Samhita*. Thanks to the Yale medical and university libraries, an original and highly detailed English translation in four volumes has provided the backbone for the present work (Kaviratna, 1902–1925). The current text, it is hoped, will bring Ayurveda into contemporary focus and help advance a proper and more formal recognition of this "life wisdom" that will auspiciously facilitate its achieving status as a significant part of world medicine for the third millennium.

May 2000
New Haven, Connecticut

CHAPTER 1

BACKGROUND, HISTORY, AND DEVELOPMENT

AYURVEDA WITHIN THE CONTEXT OF WORLD CULTURE

Lord Dhanvantari was regarded, in ancient India, as the deity or patron of classical medicine. He continues to hold that honor among Ayurvedic physicians today. Most depictions and statuary show him holding in his left hand a bowl of *amrit*, the nectar of life; his right hand holds a medical text, an herb, a leech, and a knife. These items, symbolizing the whole range of medicine and surgery, serve as a model of inspiration spanning past and present. The opening passages of the *Sushruta Samhita* (Acharya & Pandurang, 1945; Bhishagratna, 1968; Trikamji & Ram, 1980), an ancient Indian medical text, describe Ayurveda's mythological origins in the following way:

> "O, Sire, it grieves us much to find men, though otherwise well befriended by their kin and relations, falling prey to diseases, mental, physical, coming to them from outside or from their inner being, and piteously wailing in agony like utterly friendless creatures on earth; and we supplicate thee, O Lord, to illumine our minds with the truths of the Eternal Ayurveda so that we may faithfully discharge the duties allotted to us in life, and alleviate the sufferings of humanity at large. Bliss in this life and hereafter is in the gift of this eternal Ayurveda, and for this, O Lord, we have made bold to approach thee as thy humble disciples." To them thus replied the holy Dhanvantari, "Welcome to all of you to this blissful hermitage. All of you are worthy of the honor of true pupilship or tutelage."

Ayurveda is a Sanskrit word meaning the knowledge, wisdom, or science of life in the sense of the optimal measure of all aspects of high-quality and healthy living. It has its origins in the distant past before the historical period of written documentation and is believed to have been formulated by the ancient sages (*rishis*) of India who were considered individuals with the stature of mental giants. The accurate dating of the historical origins of Ayurveda, like that of traditional Chinese medicine, is uncertain. Dating, therefore, may be considered only an approximation, in part derived from surviving documents, and in larger measure from tradition. Historical accuracy becomes more objectively verifiable during and after the advent of Buddhism in the sixth century B.C., and with the historical writings of the Greek historian, Herodotus (c. 490 / 80–425 B.C.). His commentaries, especially on the Greek and Persian wars, reflect a very active international exchange of conflict, conquest, and ideas.

The significance of this documented, early (c. 550 B.C.) contact between Persia and Greece lies in the fact that the Persian empire constituted the geographical, if not cultural, link between India and territories to the west—the Near East and the Roman Empire. The ancestors of the Persians were derived, in part, from the same Aryan peoples who, it is believed, brought the Vedas, ancient wisdom texts, to India in the second millennium B.C. (Biardeau, 1989). In addition, Cyrus the Great captured Babylon in 539 B.C. This conquest gave Persia control over Mesopotamia and the entire Babylonian Empire that then reached to the borders of Egypt. Historical sources testify to the fact that the Persian Empire, at this early date, borrowed heavily from the cultures of Assyria, Babylonia, Egypt, and Greece. To what extent Persia absorbed parts of India's culture and Ayurveda is not clearly documented. Some Indian influence may have occurred and contributed to the development of Persian medicine. An Ayurvedic influence becomes clearer much later, and is reflected in the prolific work of the Persian physician Avicenna in the 10th century A.D.

After Cyrus, the subsequent Persian ruler, Darius (c. 522 B.C.) entered India (Figure 1.1) and annexed the Sind (the ancient Mohenjo-daro area) and, perhaps, the Punjab region (ancient Harappa). Later, Alexander the Great (c. 334 B.C.) not only conquered the Persians, but in 327 B.C., entered India, and there

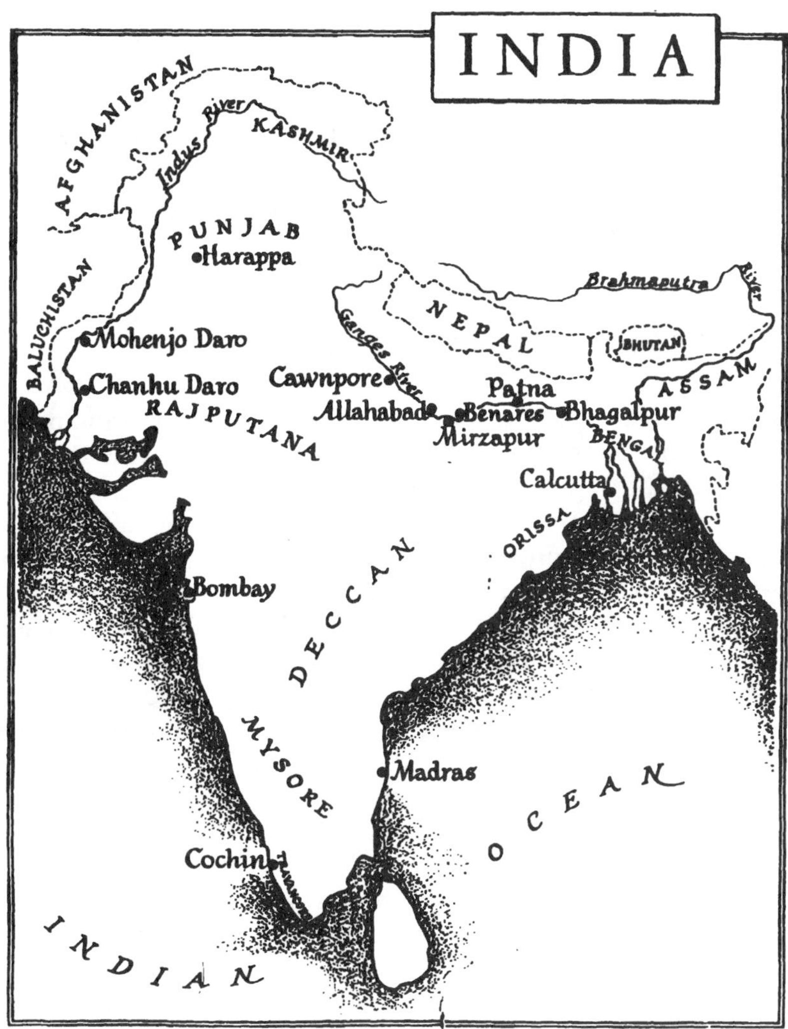

Figure 1.1. Map of ancient India with older names of cities and regions. Mohenjo-daro was in the Sind region. Harappa was in the Punjab region. Ancient Taxila was on the Indus river, north of Harappa in the Kashmir region, now modern Pakistan. The Hindu Kush pass was northwest of Harappa. Benares was also called Varanasi. (From *A History of Medicine, Vol. 2: Early Greek, Hindu, and Persian Medicine* by Henry E. Sigerist, copyright © 1961, 1987 by Oxford University Press, Inc. Used by permission of Oxford University Press.)

defeated the Indian king Poros. Aspects of Hellenic culture, therefore, were introduced into India and some aspects of Indian culture including Ayurveda were surely absorbed by the Greeks and Persians. Bloodshed and an active need for medical and surgical skill no doubt accompanied these invasions and military conflicts. The exchange of medicosurgical knowledge between the cultures—India, the Middle East, and the Greek and Roman West—especially via this route, is an implied certainty (Wohlberg, 1990).

WRITTEN HISTORY AND ORAL TRADITION

The primitive roots of culture are believed to have formally developed just after the last Ice Age (c. 10,000 B.C.). This first occurred in the region of the Near East. The transition from a hunter–gatherer lifestyle to an agricultural one with a food-producing economy contributed to stability over time in a central geographical location. Jericho, near present-day Jerusalem, was the site of the Natufian culture (c. 9500 B.C.). The area called Catal-Huyuk in present-day Turkey was the home of another complex Neolithic culture (c. 8500 B.C.). These two areas were focal points of agriculture and the domestication of animals by 7000 B.C. Hallmarks of civilization include literacy, organized religion, art forms, stable settlements and planned cities, agriculture, and the domestication of animals. The Mesopotamian city of Sumer is considered the first recognizable city, its origins dating back to the fourth millennium B.C. The earliest known writing is early Mesopotamian cuneiform and dates to about 3300 B.C.

Formal history begins with the written word. Written documents in various formats began to appear about the middle of the fourth millennium B.C. with hieroglyphic, cuneiform, and Minoan script. Significant medical content can be found in early writings such as the *Rig-Veda* of India (presumed origin c. 1500 B.C.), the *Codex Hammurabi* of Mesopotamia (c. 1755 B.C.), and the *Medical Papyrus Ebers* of Egypt (1570 B.C.) (Sigerist, 1951).

A legacy of written documents describing the medical systems of these eras is sorely lacking in current times. They are either undiscovered or nonexistent. Scholarship, in the form of libraries dedicated to collections of writings that reflect the history, literature, art, and science of the times, appears to have been launched in ancient Assyria when Ashurbanipal amassed the most complete collection available at the time in his grand library of Ninivah (c. 647 B.C.). It is inferred that this included not only local contributions but also the scientific, literary, and artistic writings that were taken from his conquest of Egypt. Ptolemy I (c. 305 B.C.) later brought together arguably the greatest and most complete library of its time in Alexandria, Egypt. Perganum (c. 200 B.C.) in Asia Minor was the site of another library said to rival that of Alexandria with an especially impressive Hellenistic influence gathered from the Roman conquests of Syracuse (c. 212 B.C.) and later of Corinth (c. 146 B.C.). Of importance is the fact that these early library collections, especially in Alexandria, with all their probable historical masterpieces were progressively destroyed beginning in 47 B.C. when Caesar was compelled to set fire to his fleet to prevent its falling into the hands of the Egyptians. What remained of the library was destroyed in piecemeal fashion at various later periods, according to historical tradition, probably culminating around 642 A.D. with the capture of Alexandria by the Muslims.

Ayurveda, sometimes referred to as Indian medical science, has its origins in the *Rig-Veda* and later Vedas, particularly the *Athara-Veda* (presumed origin c. 1200 B.C.). These roots suggest that Ayurveda may be among the oldest systematized forms of medicine, and subsequently may have contributed to or influenced later medical systems both in Asia and in the West. Ayurveda's origins lie in an oral tradition. Verifiable, written documentation is sparse and relies heavily on the Vedas, a group of religious and philosophical writings, and particularly the oldest one, the *Rig-Veda*. *Veda* is the Sanskrit word meaning science, knowledge, or wisdom. *Rig* is a Sanskrit word that connotes "stanzas of praise." Historians have found it almost impossible to date the Vedic hymns and poetry with any degree of accuracy. Their content is known to have been transmitted by word of mouth for centuries, if not millennia, before they were written down. In a similar fashion, historians acknowledge that the *Iliad* and *Odyssey* of ancient Greece were sung by itinerant bards long before they were edited and collected in the form known to us today. The oldest known manuscript of the Vedic scriptures dates to the 15th century A.D. Its actual origins, however, are believed to be much older, and archaeological evidence demonstrates that these writings, in fact, do reflect aspects of the earliest Indus civilization (c. 2500–1750 B.C.).

INDIAN CULTURE

Ayurveda and Indian culture are inseparably linked (Kak, 1987). By about 2500 B.C. and before 1500 B.C., India was mainly inhabited by the Dravidians, an indigenous, dark-skinned people about whose origins little is known. The forebears of these varied groups of tribal cultures are thought to have come from the earlier Neolithic cultures (7000–6000 B.C.) of Afghanistan and Baluchistan to the northwest. These peoples, also referred to as the pre-Harappan or Early Indus culture, established complex urban sites in northwest India along the Indus River. It is inferred that these peoples had an already developed culture with significant material, psychological, and spiritual dimensions. This civilization reached its peak around 2300 B.C. and trade links with Mesopotamia have been dated to this period. The culture of the mature Indus or Harappan civilization is seen in the regions called Mohenjo-daro in Sind and Harappa in Punjab (Dales & Kenoyer, 1993). These areas have yielded impressive archaeological finds, and are recognized as the most important and extensive Bronze Age sites. Their hieroglyphic style of writing has yet to be deciphered (Parpola, 1994). Material evidence from these sites suggests a strong cultural unity, evidence of trading links with Mesopotamia, and a high degree of uniformity of urban planning. The high level of sophistication of these cultures is solidly demonstrated by their meticulously organized city planning with complex drainage systems, the earliest known evidence of cotton cultivation, and a standardized system of weights and measures in use for commerce. Mohenjodaro is recognized as one of the oldest, if not the oldest, known planned city. Significant material evidence from this very early period is highly suggestive of a cultural recognition of a spiritual dimension with religious overtones. Figurines and steatite seals having god and goddesslike images have been uncovered. The famous Pasupati seal has been inferred to possibly represent a prototype of the Hindu god, Shiva, the yogin and Lord of the animals, having three faces and siting in a classic Yoga posture. This Indus and pre-Aryan culture, therefore, is thought to contain early and important elements of what later developed into the Vedic tradition.

Sometime in the second millennium B.C., a new group of people, who are thought to have come from the plains of central Asia, came into northwest India through the passes of the Hindu Kush (Fairservis, 1975). This fair-skinned race, the Aryans, meaning "noble" or "wise," is associated with the decline of the previous Indus civilization. Their language was Vedic Sanskrit, one of the oldest Indo-European root languages. They brought the sacred scriptures, the Vedas, into India. The Vedas reflect a total worldview that includes aspects of creation, metaphysics, philosophy, ethics, religion, magic, medicine, dietary rules, and guidelines for the activities of daily living. The Aryan culture (1500–500 B.C.) is believed to have merged with and dominated the pre-Aryan peoples of the Indus civilization. Although the Aryans exerted an overriding influence on the developing culture, including religion and philosophy, of India during this period, the earlier indigenous Dravidians, especially in central and southern India, the Deccan and Mysore regions, made important and substantial contributions to the form and content of this newly emerging Aryan evolution. Recent speculation has proposed a more intimate link between Dravidian and Aryan cultures, if not an actual identity.

THE ANCIENT VEDAS

The Aryans who brought the Vedas or cannons of wisdom into India considered them the foundation of their culture and way of life. To this day, the Vedas are still considered by orthodox Hindus to be the most authoritative source and template of all knowledge (Zaehner, 1966; Zimmer, 1951). They were believed to have been revealed by the godhead, Brahma, creator of the universe, and received, in fact, heard (*sruti*) by inspired sages (*rishis*) who passed them on by word of mouth. Sages were leaders of extraordinary wisdom having the unique quality of *apta* (inspiration and authority). The Vedas, four in number, therefore, have a twofold denotation that encompasses both revelation (*sruti*), whose content is not of human origin (*apaurusya*), and, as well, the literature reflecting this sacred knowledge that was written down many centuries later. The Vedas are considered to have been composed around 1500 to 1200 B.C.; this dating regarding their oral compilation is a conservative and generally accepted idea. Others speculate that the Vedas were received by the *rishis* much earlier, possibly 3000 B.C. or even earlier but finally redacted around 1500 B.C. The standard Vedic form for the teaching, learning, and dissemination of the Vedas and the subsequent commentaries on them, in fact, consisted of their being sung as hymns or *sutras* (aphorisms in the form of oral prose / poetry). Pupils sat across from the teacher (*up-pa-sad*) and, in an intimately solemn and interpersonal fashion, recited the sutras of knowledge and wisdom.

The guardians and disseminators of the Vedas were the priestly class called *Brahmins*. The Brahmanic tradition is virtually synonymous with the Vedic tradition. Written versions of some Vedic commentaries appeared relatively late, around the middle of the first millennium B.C. The Vedas, therefore, constituted an oral body of knowledge that was transmitted from generation to generation but not organized into written form until well into the second millennium A.D. The profound significance of the Vedas lies in their being the bedrock upon which Ayurveda rests. The continuity of this ancient relationship is clearly suggested by a recognized tradition that regards Ayurveda as an *upaveda* or supplementary Veda, with some going so far as to reverently ascribe to it the standing the "fifth Veda."

The primary Vedas are the four mantric or hymnal texts: the *Rig-Veda*, the *Yajur-Veda*, the *Sama-Veda*, and the *Athara-Veda*. The *Rig-Veda* (Griffith, 1973; O'Flaherty, 1981) is considered the oldest and is reputedly the source of the other three. It is made up of stanzas of adulation (*rik*) that are compiled in 10 books (*mandala*), which contain 1,028 sacred mantras, chants, hymns, and verses. Ayurvedic tradition, as well as some scholarly speculation, suggests that its content reflects events occurring earlier than 6000 B.C. The *Sama-Veda* (Ganapati, 1992) contains 1,810 mantras developed into musical forms, songs (*saman*), priestly chants, and instructions on their recitation. The *Yajur-Veda* contains action or ritual formulas (*yajus*) especially composed for sacrificial rites. It consists of five *samhitas*, collections of prayers and ritual texts in verse and prose. The *Athara-Veda* (Bloomfield, 1967; Dwight, 1984; Whitney & Lanman, 1996) contains 731 magical incantations and ritual texts with a preponderance of medically related information spanning 20 books, and is the Veda most closely associated with later Ayurvedic texts. The *Athara-Veda* may have been composed around 1200 B.C. Many diseases are mentioned, including fever, diarrhea, heart disease, jaundice, cough, leprosy, and mania. In addition, there are ample references to obstetric and gynecological issues and procedures as well as to what we now recognize as mental disorders. Later authoritative supplements and appendixes based on the primary Vedic collections (*samhitas*) were called *Brahmanas* (ritual texts), *Aranyakas* (forest texts), and *Upanishads* (self-development spiritual texts) (Bedekar & Palsule, 1995; Radhakrishnan, 1953). These writings developed the ideas contained in the *samhitas* and are considered to be part of the primary Vedic corpus. This ancient Vedic medicine, like Greek archaic medicine, had religious and magic elements. Certainly, no early Greek texts comparable to the *Athara-Veda* have come down to us, perhaps because there were none or because of the destruction of the libraries in ancient Alexandria that may have housed them. The Vedas remain repositories of principles of understanding that are heavily suffused with moral precepts and rules of conduct. The Vedas, therefore, stand as an extant grand monument at the very beginning of Indian literature presenting a record of what is believed to be the source of all knowledge, including medicine and science.

Since the Vedic period (c. 1500 to 500 B.C.) may be considered the foundation not only of Indian culture but also of Ayurveda, some significant aspects of the Vedic worldview as expressed in daily life will be addressed. Two of the most central themes around which Vedic culture was organized were that of the significance of *fire* and that of *ritual sacrifice* (Heesterman, 1993; Staal, 1983). It may be difficult for modern man to fully appreciate the centrality that the phenomenon of fire had almost 6,000 years ago. Not only was basic survival predicated on it, but the maturation and development of civilization was also enhanced. Fire provided warmth, the ability to cook and use a variety of foods (predominantly milk, ghee, grains, and meats), sterilization of water and foods, purification and cleaning, and light by which to extend human activities into the night. Man, at that time, was dependent on fire for survival. The singular importance of fire was expressed in the Vedic reification of it. Fire was identified with the god *Agni.* The conceptual understanding of *Agni* was multilayered. It included associations with heat, the sun, part of the earth as the sacred cow, *Prisni,* with the digestive fire within the human stomach, and as being the actual fire used in sacrificial ritual. The profound significance, meaning, and value of fire to humans and their well-being in the ancient world can be equated in meaning and significance to that of electricity in the modern world.

The concept of ritual and sacrifice is an ancient one (Jamison, 1991; Vesci, 1992). Its meaning includes a ritualized process whereby man gives offerings to a higher or transcendent reality. The concept of prayer is implicit in this activity. The idea that this may result in some beneficial effect is implied but complex. By the fifth century B.C., Vedic society had an established set of guidelines that charted out a developmental sequence of life stages (*asramas*) especially for the priestly classes. The second stage entailed obligations set by the mandates of prescribed dharmic responsibilities to establish a strong central and extended traditional family unit within which a variety of intricate home-based and public-based rituals were regularly performed. For the Brahmanic priests in Vedic times, sacrifice or *homa* consisted of a ritual sequence in which a material substance such as milk, ghee, yogurt, rice, barley, an animal, or the sacred plant, *Soma,* was put into a sacred fire and immolated wholly or in part. In addition, parts of the sacrificial offering were consumed by the participants and parts were believed to be consumed by the gods (*devas*) or transcendent forces invoked. The oldest Vedic literature makes clear that ritual sacrifice is a mandate of *dharma,* the natural law of the Vedic universe that sets categorical imperatives for man but does not include an explicit promise of reward. Ritual sacrifice was a human obligation done for ritual's sake alone. Acknowledgment, awe, and praise appear to have been an integral part of the mindset of those performing these obligatory, daily duties. The Western conception of the meaning of prayer has similar features.

The Vedic concept of sacrifice, however, remains complex in its subtleties (Staal, 1989). Having no expectation of reward was considered a virtue in fulfilling one's life choices or *dharma* in the formal Vedic literature (pre 500 B.C.). Post-Vedic literature, moreover, and commentaries on the Vedic *samhitas*, expanded and extended this initial conception. One may speculate that some of the significant motivations and intentions behind the act of sacrifice reflected a psychological posture that included aspects of deference, remembrance, renewal, and gratitude. The one that engaged in the ritual sacrifice was called the *yajamana*. His actions indicated an awareness of a transcendent reality that required recognition. This strongly connotes a sense of another and is characterized by a mood of awe and reverence; in fact, this may be termed a sense of the *sacred* or the *spiritual*. This implies a level of cognitive expansion able to abstract immaterial themes, i.e., meaning, from concrete, literal, and material experience.

One outstanding feature of Vedic ritual, however, was that of fostering remembrance (*smirti*) considered an antidote to the natural inclination to forget. Remembrance and a conscious awareness of the Vedic worldview are enhanced by the continued recognition of *dharma's* rules, laws, personal and social obligations, values, and virtues. The Vedic sacrificial ritual consisted of a material offering into the sacred fire accompanied by the recitations of several Brahmanic priests who spoke and chanted Vedic axioms from the four major Vedas. Mandates concerning ritual, sacrifice, and lawful behavior were made explicit. The experience of the sacrificial ritual, a solemn liturgy of action and the recounting of Vedic law, done in a communal setting, reinforced remembrance on a daily and repeated basis.

The central intention behind sacrificial acts was to express the fundamental Vedic belief in the nexus between microcosm as man and macrocosm as universe. This cosmic homology was a fundamental Vedic theme. The Vedas rigorously adhered to the idea of man's need to preserve his harmony and alignment with the rest of nature. This coordination or correspondence was termed *bandhu* and was mediated by the transformative power of *Agni*. The sacrificial fires, by their innate powers, resulted in the acquisition of purity, health, auspiciousness, grace, and a regulation of any imbalances created by man both within himself and in the world. Ritual sacrifice, therefore, was considered vital; as such, it was organized in daily life around the natural cycles of the 24–hour period, the junctures of seasons, the cycle of the moon, and the chronological life cycle from birth to death. The observance of ritual and sacrifice, therefore, had several axiomatic themes: remembrance, ongoing need for purification, and the dharmic mandate to uphold the integrity of the human and extended universe.

The intimate identity between the ritual sacrifical fire, *Agni*, and the digestive fire became explicit in later Upanishad commentaries and was acknowledged early on in the work of the Ayurvedic physicians, *Charaka* and *Sushruta* (c. 700 B.C.). The medical reality and practical significance of this was an essential part of Ayurveda in ancient times and, in essence, continues today. In modern times, the transmutational dynamic of ancient ritual sacrificial action is reflected in a recognition of one's duty to observe dietary and lifestyle practices that foster and optimize the transformative action of *Agni*, the digestive metabolism in the body. Paralleling what had been ritual and sacrificial duties in the past are activities practiced now in more sublimated forms: study of the ancient writings, meditation, and acts that reflect a sense of gratitude, reconciliation, and harmony between man and the greater world of which he is part. These all contribute to the theory and practice of Ayurveda in contemporary times.

The *Rig-Veda*, therefore, considered one of the oldest extant compilations reflecting the daily life of an ancient civilization, attests to a life-affirming, awe-filled celebration of all that is earthy and material. These ancient canons show that this ancient culture experienced all aspects of the world in tangible ways using visual acuity, a developed sense of sound, tactile awareness, olfactory sensation, and taste. Every sense organ of these ancient peoples savored in reverence the experience of the senses as they interacted with the material world around. At this early Vedic period, nowhere is found any indication of a sense of renunciation of the physical world or of its being qualitatively subordinate to anything else. There is a simultaneous poignant awareness of a spiritual dimension, demonstrated by pervasive ritual and sacrifice. This, however, is not displayed in a delimited or circumscribed fashion. The spiritual aspect of Vedic life, an awareness of a consciousness intrinsic in nature and of powers having limited but possible access to humans, imbues all activities of daily living. It is this wide and all-encompassing perspective that echoes throughout the origins and development of the ancient Vedic worldview and finds current expression in Ayurveda today.

THE CLASSICAL EPIC AND PURANIC PERIODS

The Vedic period ended about 500 B.C. Subsequent texts deriving from the primary Vedic *samhitas* laid more emphasis on the *dharma* of self-development but with more explicit spiritual, mystical, and philosophical content (Hiltebeitel, 1999). These writings, commentaries, and interpretations of the Vedas are known as *Vedanta,* meaning "end of the Vedas." The important subgroup known as the Upanishads (c. 600 B.C.–A.D. 1600) has the distinction of containing original metaphysical contributions that antedate even the beginnings of Greek philosophy. It is considered the primary source Vedanta upon which later Vedantists further elaborated. Other significant texts, considered, however, of secondary importance to the Vedas, were in the form of epic poems. The *Ramayana,* the *Mahabharata,* and the *Bhagavad Gita,* a section of the *Mahabharata,* were first written down during the Vedanta period but, like the Vedas, appear to be set much earlier, between 1000 and 700 B.C. (Buitenen, 1973–1978, 1981; Johnson, 1994; Narasimhan, 1997; Prabhupada, 1997). Further significant contributions to Vedanta were made by Shankara (A.D. 788–820), Ramanuja (A.D. 1017–1137), and

Madhva (c. A.D. 1238), all of whom are considered major spiritual figures in Indian culture. The foundations of Indian philosophy, religion, and culture are rooted in these ancient works. Mention should be made of an important group of literature called *Puranas*. They were written from about A.D. 320 through A.D. 520 and have been continuously amended up to Medieval times (c. A.D. 1500). These "stories of the ancient past" are narratives that contain genealogies of deities and kings, cosmologies, law codes, descriptions of rituals, and pilgrimages to holy places. These expositions related specific details of religious systems that centered on deities such as Vishnu, Shiva, and Devi. Devi is also known as *Shakti* and is considered the feminine consort of Shiva. This last classical period produced much of what constitutes India's current and diverse contemporary spiritual sects (Kripal, 1998; Lipner, 1994; Narang, 1984; Oberoi, 1995; Sivaraman, 1973).

THE DEVELOPMENT OF EARLY MEDICINE AND AYURVEDA

Evidence shows that scientific or rational medicine, as it exists today, had its beginnings in Greece with the school of Hippocrates in the fifth century B.C. (Sigerist, 1961). Before that, the main streams of the healing arts came from Minoan culture (2200–1450 B.C.), Egyptian culture (2700 B.C.), the Indus Valley / Harappan culture (2500–1700 B.C.), and the Mesopotamian / Babylonian priestly tradition (2300 B.C.). Ayurvedic medicine, as it began to appear in written form, owes a great debt to the advent of Buddhism in the sixth century B.C. Many great Ayurvedic physicians became Buddhists and many Buddhist monks began to chronicle the development of Ayurveda within India and later in foreign lands such as Ceylon (Sri Lanka), Tibet, and China, paralleling their missionary excursions.

AYURVEDA AND BUDDHISM

During the lifetime of the Buddha (c. 563–483 B.C.) and for a time thereafter, Indian culture experienced a Golden Age of development during which learning and trade expanded until the 12th century A.D. when Muslim forces entered India and ruled until about 1700. The development of Buddhism and that of Ayurveda became closely entwined (Clifford, 1984). Ayurveda emerged out of the ancient Vedas and retained allegiance to its authority as did most developing Indian systems, much later referred to as *Hindu*. Buddhism, however, perhaps in an attempt to purify, restructure, or reform the older Vedic traditions, in effect, appeared to abandon them, at least concerning their detailed ritualistic mandates. Buddhism, moreover, was comfortable adopting Ayurveda as a medical and therapeutic program. During the fifth to fourth centuries B.C., the University at Taxila, north of ancient Harappa, whose present site is modern Pakistan, was a major node of higher learning. Jivaka, one of Taxila's outstanding Ayurvedic physicians, was the royal doctor and son of king Bimbisara of the kingdom of Magadha south of the Ganges river in northeast India and he was also Buddha's personal physician. Jivaka is reputed to have been expert in many subspecialties of medicine and a variety of surgical techniques. He was considered the most skilled physician of his time, and stories about his achievements abounded in all the Buddhist territories, namely Magadha in northeast India, Benares, and Peshawar near the Khyber Pass (between modern western Pakistan and Afghanistan) in northern Asia near China.

The association between Buddhist doctrine, with its emphasis on moral and ethical behavior, and its espousal of Ayurveda became renowned during this time. It led king Ashoka, emperor of most of northern India, to become a convert to Buddhism in the third century B.C. Ayurvedic medicine became widely disseminated through this ruler's establishment of a number of charitable hospitals with extensive medical, surgical, and psychiatric components to treat both humans and animals. This reflected the pragmatic implementation of the Buddhist virtue of compassion for all sentient beings. There are extant documents cut in rock that display Ashoka's edicts directing embassies to be erected in foreign lands and ordering Buddhist missionaries to travel within and outside of India to disseminate the teachings. It is believed that Ayurveda and Theravada Buddhism, an early Buddhist perspective that laid great emphasis on renunciation, self-discipline, and individual self-development outside of mainstream society, reached Sri Lanka at this time. The Bower Manuscript, written in the fourth century A.D., that was found in Central Asia attests to the fact that Buddhist medical missionary work continued and expanded at this time. The introduction of Ayurveda into Tibet took place around A.D. 650 with the translation of Buddhist Ayurvedic texts into Tibetan. The history of the spread of Buddhism throughout the East, therefore, may be seen as paralleling the expansion and impact that Ayurveda had outside of its home in India.

ANCIENT AYURVEDIC MEDICAL TEXTS: *CHARAKA SAMHITA, SUSHRUTA SAMHITA*

The *Charaka Samhita* (Kaviratna, 1902–1925; Mehta, 1949; Ray & Gupta, 1965; Sharma, 1995), a major Ayurvedic compendium of medical theory and practice, may have been formulated around 1000 B.C. or earlier, but is believed to have been redacted by the famous Ayurvedic physician Charaka of Kashmir, at the University of Taxila, and compiled in written form around 760 B.C. It is uncertain whether this organized medical collection was the work of one man or the school of Charaka's followers. This *samhita* was composed in the form of prose and poetry with over 8,400 verses in eight major sections and 120 lessons or chapters. These were memorized and lyrically recited by Ayurvedic physicians of ancient times and continue to be recited to this day by modern Ayurvedic physicians. Charaka discusses the field of internal medicine, describes the five subdoshas of *Vata* (the five bioenergetic, physiological principles that regulate the central nervous system and all movements in the body), and gives particular emphasis to the value, care, and priority of the consciousness within man. Of particular note, given the lack of the microscope at that early time, are Charaka's detailed descriptions of anatomical dissection and analysis of skin with enumeration of its six layers.

Sushruta of Varanasi (Benares), a great Ayurvedic surgeon, produced the other classic medicosurgical text, the *Sushruta Samhita,* around 660 B.C. (Acharya & Pandurang, 1945; Bhishagratna, 1968; Trikamji & Ram, 1980). This *samhita,* composed in both prose and poetry, emphasized a surgical viewpoint. The importance of blood is extensively addressed. Sushruta includes the first description of the five subdoshas of *Pitta* (the five bioenergetic, physiological principles that regulate the body's metabolic functioning), and gives a classic definition of the concept of health. Like Charaka, using only the naked eye, he goes on to describe the layers of the skin. Together, the *Charaka Samhita* and the *Sushruta Samhita* are considered the oldest extant classic texts of Ayurvedic medicine and surgery. These two medical compendia constitute the historically documented foundations of most of Ayurvedic medicine. Modern medicine today recognizes some of the ancient Indian roots of current medical and surgical practice (Das, 1984; Kansupada & Sassani, 1997; Prakash, 1978; Savithri, 1987). Inhalation therapy can be traced back to India some 4,000 years ago (Grossman, 1994). Sushruta has been called the father of surgery since he was the first to develop acknowledgedly novel techniques in plastic and reconstructive surgery such as the use of skin grafts and procedures for total nasal reconstruction (Hauben, Baruchin, & Mahler, 1982; Nichter, Morgan, & Nichter, 1983). A timeline of the Ayurvedic oral and written tradition will be found in Appendix 1.

A SHORT HISTORY OF WESTERN MEDICINE AND AYURVEDA

Hippocrates (460 B.C.) is considered the father of Western medicine (Porter, 1997; Singer & Underwood, 1962). His methods, unlike those of his predecessors, were less influenced by animist and other religious doctrines. He is reputed to have relied more on detailed clinical observation and to have had closer clinical contact when evaluating and treating individual patients. The school of Hippocrates held the humoral theory in which the body was believed to be composed of four *humors*: blood (*sanguis*), phlegm (*pituita*), yellow bile (*chole*), and black bile (*melanchole*). Humors were considered to be vaporous material substances contributing to health as well as being capable of going awry and causing illness. This notion was applied clinically to delineate constitutional and temperamental body types.

Dietary therapy and the influence of the seasons on health and disease were also very prominent features of the Hippocratic tradition. To what extent these theories and practices were influenced by the much older yet very similar Ayurvedic concepts remains unknown.

Aristotle (384 B.C.), the great codifier of ancient science, using a perspective similar to that of Hippocrates, relied heavily on empirical observation and naturalistic classification. An important part of his ontology and taxonomy was a classification system using what he referred to as the four *prime qualities*: hot, cold, wet, and dry, together with four fundamental *essences* or *elements*: air, fire, water, and earth. Emphasis was placed more on anatomical description rather than physiological functioning. As with Hippocrates' use of the humors and constitutional types, Aristotle's descriptive and explanatory use of the *qualities* and *elements* is strikingly similar to those found in the historically older Ayurvedic concepts.

When Alexander the Great invaded India in 327 B.C. and temporarily occupied the Sind and Punjab areas, historical reports describe his contact with Ayurvedic physicians whose talents he is said to have used almost exclusively to treat poisoning cases in his armies. It is plausible to believe that he and his cohort of physicians took some of this Ayurvedic knowledge back to the West, perhaps influencing the then early development of the Greek medical corpus.

Galen of Pergamon (A.D. 129–215) was an influential physician in the Western Latin world, especially in Rome. He is reputed to have been trained in Asia Minor and at the medical school in Alexandria, Egypt. The substance of his work was derived from the *Corpus Hippocraticum*, a collection of medical writings that have been transmitted through the ages and attributed to Hippocrates and his school. The form of Galen's practice was taken from the Aristotelian method. He held a rationalist view placing reason, observation, and experimentation over knowledge derived from empirical or sense-based experience. Via the Arabic tradition that developed later, Galen became the most influential physician of the ancient world. His distinctively Western style then became the theoretical basis for all of Western medical practice for the next 1500 years until the 16th century

A.D. Indeed, his influence persisted until the end of the 19th century in spite of the discoveries of 17th-century medicine, such as Harvey's description of the circulation of the blood in 1615 and van Leeuwenhoek's microscopic observations of cells and microbes (c. 1700).

CHINESE TRADITIONAL MEDICINE AND AYURVEDA

In terms of further historical perspective, the oldest extant Chinese medical text, the *Huang-di Nei-jing* or *Inner Classic of the Yellow Emperor,* was compiled by unknown authors somewhere between 300 and 100 B.C.; some put the dating between 475 and 221 B.C. (Unschuld, 1979, 1985). There are many striking similarities in theory and clinical practice between Ayurveda and traditional Chinese medicine as well as some significant differences (Mahdihassan, 1985b, 1989; Wiseman & Ellis, 1985). The influence of Ayurveda, perhaps brought to China by itinerant, missionary Indian Buddhist monks, has been suggested.

Historically, there is evidence that the Chinese Yueh-chih tribes, the Kushans, coming from western China, occupied Benares (Varanasi) in northeast India. They are considered to have formed a bridge, in effect, between East and West, traversing the Silk Road. The Burma Road (115 B.C.) to the south also opened the exchange of material goods and ideas to and from China. Trade with the Roman Empire, at the height of its wealth, included spices, ivory, and other luxuries. The third and greatest Kushan king, Kanishka (c. A.D. 100), whose capital was Peshawar near the Khyber Pass close to ancient Taxila, was considered to be a great patron of *Mahayana Buddhism,* the system that fosters self-development through compassion within a social context. He ushered its entry into northern Asia and China. Records show that Buddhist monasteries were established in China by A.D. 65 and that there existed translations of Sanskrit texts into Chinese in the Luoyang region by the second century A.D. (Chen, 1984). From China, Buddhism then spread to Korea in the fourth century and to Japan in the sixth century. The Ayurvedic influence, since it existed in tandem with Buddhism for so many centuries, may have contributed to traditional Chinese medicine by this association.

NAGARJUNA: BUDDHIST PRIEST, PHILOSOPHER, AND AYURVEDIC PHYSICIAN

The development of Ayurveda, particularly in regard to its medicinal armamentarium, was further advanced by the great Buddhist priest, philosopher, and Ayurvedic physician, Nagarjuna, around A.D. 100 (Garfield, 1995; Hajicek-Dobberstein, 1995; Kalupahana, 1986; Lindtner, 1997; Mahdihassan, 1981, 1985a; Sharma, 1977; White, 1996; Williams, 1989). He is considered the father of *iatrochemistry,* the science of the preparation of medicinal mineral substances. Up to this time, most medical interventions of the Charaka tradition were derived from an herbal or plant-based pharmacopoeia, while Ayurvedic physicians of the Sushruta School were more skilled in surgical approaches. Nagarjuna's effort was to expand the therapeutic armamentarium by constructing a mineral-based repertoire of active, healing substances. Many heretofore toxic substances, like mercury, were now processed in complex ways, using the innovative techniques of the Nagarjuna School, to render them nontoxic and suitable for human consumption. This opened a new and much broader field for development and expanded the range of therapeutic interventions that today continue to be an integral and characteristic aspect of Ayurvedic medicine. The brilliance of Nagarjuna's contributions, however, extended far beyond this and encompassed a qualitative advance in Buddhist theory and practice with an especially productive literature both in medicine as well as philosophy and religion.

During the fourth century A.D., the Buddhists, who excelled in both intellectual and practical endeavors, set up the renowned university of Nalanda in the region of Bihar, northwest India near Patna. It retained its prominence until the 12th century. Some of the subjects taught included history, geography, literature, law, mathematics, trade, commerce, and medicine. There are descriptions in the historical archives by Chinese travelers telling of the university's diverse culture and commenting on the estimated 10,000 students and 1,500 teachers who were involved in academic pursuits.

ASHTANGA: AYURVEDIC MEDICAL TEXTS OF VAGBHATA

The seventh century produced another great Ayurvedic scholar and Buddhist, *Vagbhata* of Sind, in northwest India. His effort and that of his followers produced the next greatest collection of Ayurvedic medical writings, the *Ashtanga Sagraha,* and about 100 years later, the collection known as the *Ashtanga Hridhaya* (Harishastri, 1939; Moos, 1984). The *Sagraha* is primarily composed in the form of poetry; the *Hridhaya* is in prose. Within these works, the first description of the five subdoshas of *Kapha* (the five bioenergetic, physiological principles that regulate and contribute to the body's structure and physical form) is presented. This significant text gave emphasis to the more material value of life than that found in Charaka and Sushruta. Even today, the *Ashtanga Hridhaya* is highly regarded as a primary medical text by the Ayurvedic physicians in Kerala, southern India. The triune of texts, *Charaka Samhita, Sushruta Samhita,* and the *Ashtangas* of Vagbhata is referred to as the *Brihat Trayi,* the senior or greater triad. These three works are universally recognized as the textual foundations of Ayurvedic medicine.

THE ARAB MEDICAL TRADITION OF AVICENNA

The parallel progress of medicine can also be seen in the work of the Persian physician *Avicenna* (A.D. 980–1037). He produced the comprehensive *Canon of Medicine,* a compendium of the previous works of Hippocrates and Galen. It was to become the preeminent medical text for both the Muslim world and the entire Latin West until the 17th century. Arab or Muslim medicine had been and continues to be known as *Unani Tibb* (Greek-based medicine) which connotes the very strong influence of the ancient Greek physicians on Arab medical thought. There are historical reports that describe the interchange between Ayurveda and the Middle East. Ayurvedic physicians were invited to Jundishpur and to Baghdad in the Middle East to teach and to organize hospitals. From the seventh century A.D., Arab traders along the Malabar Coast were a vehicle for the exchange of goods and ideas, including Ayurveda, between Indian and Arab cities. The great Arab physicians of the 10th and 11th centuries, Razes (died c. A.D. 923) and Avicenna (A.D. 980–1037), are thought to have had extensive knowledge of Indian medicine. Their voluminous and influential writings, incorporating Ayurvedic concepts along with those of the Greeks, were translated into Latin in the 13th century, and were used as standard medical texts in medieval Europe. Unani Tibb, for instance, holds a theory of four bodily humors and four elements. It has a constitutional typing system and uses herbal medicines in a way similar to that in Ayurveda. The influence of each system on the other seems strong.

FURTHER AYURVEDIC MEDICAL TREATISES

Between A.D. 700 and 1100, another important Ayurvedic medical text was produced, the *Madhava Nidana* (Murthy, 1987), which was devoted to a survey of diagnostic procedures with an emphasis on the classification of disease. In the 14th century, another fundamental Ayurvedic text, *Sarangadhara Samhita,* appeared. It contained the first textual reference to the unique method of Ayurvedic pulse diagnosis. A systematized materia medica with pharmacological formulations was also enumerated. In the 16th century, a final, classic, and significant text was written, the *Bhavaprakasha*. It included a description of new herbs, minerals, dietetic advances, and rejuvenation theory. Comments were also made on newly discovered sexually transmitted diseases, particularly the clinical presentation of syphilis brought into India by foreigners. This last triune of medical texts, the *Madhava Nidana,* the *Sharangadhara Samhita,* and the *Bhavaprakash* is called the *Laghu Trayi,* the junior or lesser triad of fundamental texts.

The period from the 12th to the early 18th century A.D. was dominated by Muslim control of India. This medieval period is considered an era of consolidation of Ayurvedic medicine.

Innovative developments in Ayurveda, in general, were less prominent in deference to the strong Muslim rule. Unani Tibb or Greek-based medicine prevailed, especially after the Moghul Empire was established in India in 1526.

AYURVEDA IN THE NINETEENTH AND TWENTIETH CENTURIES

The influence of Great Britain played a major role in every aspect of India's economic, social, political, and medical development (Edney, 1997). The British soldier and statesman, Robert Clive, in the service of the East India Company, in the 1750s eradicated the then dominant French influence and introduced British control. Later, around 1818, the British East India Company exerted a gradually more powerful influence that spread throughout all of India. In 1833, it closed virtually all the existing Ayurvedic training centers and schools. A British medical school was opened in Calcutta, and Western influence dominated the country, especially the medical field, for almost 100 years. In 1920 there arose a national revival and a resurgence of interest in traditional Indian culture, practices, and Ayurveda. In 1946 there was formal governmental recognition and reacceptance of Ayurveda, and a resurgence of research, development, and modernization programs.

Today, there are many Ayurvedic training schools and clinics in India. Interestingly, in India, the current belief, however, is that this traditional healing art may be unscientific according to Western standards, if not too atavistic in general. It is, therefore, relegated to a secondary place with Western or allopathic medicine in the forefront. The Indian government officially recognizes as legitimate: allopathy, homeopathy, naturopathy, Unani Tibb, Ayurveda, and its cousins, *Siddha* and *Yoga*. The Siddha system of Indian medicine is identified with those whose roots are more related to the aboriginal Dravidian culture prevalent in southern India, especially in the Tamil region. Another form of traditional medicine called *Emchi* is distinctively Tibetan and Buddhist but strongly resembles Ayurveda in theory and practice.

THE LEGENDARY ORIGINS OF AYURVEDA

While the above history has placed Ayurveda in a historical context, it also has a rich mythological history with a narrative that imparts a sense of wonder and profundity. It begins with Brahma, the creator of the universe, who is considered to be the original propounder of Ayurveda. The system, it is said, was then handed down to Daksa Prajapati, a primordial creative sage, sometimes described as a son of Brahma. From him, it was passed to the Aswin twins, considered to be divine physicians in *Swarga* or Paradise. From the Aswins, Ayurveda was handed to Indra, the supreme leader of the gods. Indra then transmitted the knowledge to his disciples: Atreya, Bharadvaja, Kasyapa, and Dhanvantari. Internal medicine was revealed primarily to Atreya Punarvasu. He conveyed it to Agnivesa, his disciple, and this culminated finally in the classical Charaka tradition.

The beginning paragraphs of the *Charaka Samhita* describe the origins of Ayurveda, the science of life, in the following way. In the most ancient of prehistoric times, a group of holy *rishis* (sages), living in the Himalayan mountains and watching over the welfare of mankind, met to discuss "the ills that flesh is heir to." The story unfolds thusly.

> When diseases arose like so many impediments to the austerity, fasting, study, continence and the vows of the embodied souls, then the great sages, the doers of good, keeping compassion for creatures foremost, met together on the sacred slopes of the Himalayas. Our body, which is the means of attaining the four aims of life, i.e., *dharma* (virtue), *artha* (worldly possessions), *kama* (pleasure), and *moksha* (liberation), is subject to diseases which emaciate and weaken it, deprive the senses of their functions, and cause extreme pain. These diseases are great impediments to our worldly affairs and bring on premature death. In the face of such enemies, how can men be happy? It is necessary, therefore, to find remedies for such diseases.

Having thus posed this seemingly insoluble and enormous dilemma, they began to meditate. In that intuitive state, they all realized that the supreme leader of all the Vedic gods, Indra, was the only authority wise enough to render an adequate solution. The first *rishi* in the assemblage to speak was Bharadvaja; he, thus, was given the mandate to approach Indra.

> Bharadvaja, the mighty ascetic, in search of (the science of) longevity approached Indra, having deemed him, the lord of the immortals, worthy of suit. Daksha Prajapati (the progenitor) first obtained the Science of Life in its entirety as promulgated by Brahma (the Great One, the Creator) and from him in turn the Ashwin twins obtained it. From the Ashwin twins the god Indra acquired it. Therefore, Bharadvaja bidden by the sages approached Indra.

Bharadvaja then disseminated this life wisdom to all the *rishis*. Atreya Punarvasu consolidated it and then transmitted it to his six disciples, one of whom was Agnivesa. It is Agnivesa's understanding that finally was synthesized into the standard medical compilation known as the *Charaka Samhita*.

The Sushruta tradition, more surgically oriented, has a complementary legendary base. The god Indra, it is said, revealed surgery to Divodasa, the King of Kasi and the city of Benares, while he was living in a hermitage. Divodasa is considered an incarnation of the god Dhanvantari, divine patron of Ayurveda. This lineage culminated finally in the classical Sushruta tradition of Ayurvedic surgery and medicine. While the school of Atreya and Bharadvaja, as mentioned previously by Charaka, specialized in general and internal medicine, the Dhanvantari School, according to Sushruta, specialized in surgery.

CHAPTER 2

THEORETICAL FOUNDATIONS AND AN OVERVIEW

> There was neither non-existence nor existence then; there was neither the realm of space nor the sky which is beyond. What stirred? Where? In whose protection? Was there water, bottomlessly deep?
>
> There was neither death nor immortality then. There was no distinguishing sign of night nor of day. That one breathed, windless, by its own impulse. Other than that there was nothing beyond.
>
> Darkness was hidden by darkness in the beginning; with no distinguishing sign, all this was water. The life force that was covered with emptiness, that one arose through the power of heat.
>
> Desire came upon that one in the beginning; that was the first seed of mind. Poets seeking in their heart with wisdom found the bond of existence in non-existence.
>
> Their cord was extended across. Was there below? Was there above? There were seed-placers; there were powers. There was impulse beneath; there was giving-forth above.
>
> Who really knows? Who will here proclaim it? Whence was it produced? Whence is this creation? The gods came afterwards, with the creation of this universe. Who then knows whence it has arisen?
>
> Whence this creation has arisen—perhaps it formed itself, or perhaps it did not—the one who looks down on it, in the highest heaven, only he knows—or perhaps he does not know [*Nasadiya*, Hymn of Creation, *Rig-Veda*, Book 10, Hymn 129; O'Flaherty, 1981, pp. 25–26].

This Vedic poetry, composed more than 4,000 years ago by the ancient sages of India, reflects the world-class profundity of their thought, imagination, and existential musings. Sages or *rishis* were considered to be of exceptional brilliance and holiness.

They were individuals who were believed to be in almost intimate contact with the divine and extraordinary dimensions of reality, and whose wisdom reflected this divine understanding, *dharma,* universal law, and divine will. Rather than advancing categorical certainties, the wisdom of the Vedas shows itself to contain a series of scholarly inquiries that are logical, empirical, erudite, and awe-inspiring. Out of the towering achievements called the Vedas, Ayurveda emerged.

There is no universally standardized Ayurvedic body of theory and clinical technique. This may be a consequence, in part, of several factors. Ayurveda is strongly clinical and empirical in application, marked by a heavy oral tradition, and has kept itself separate from the political and economic support of the times. This clinical, oral-empirical, nonlegalistic, and independent status apparently did not lend itself to a widespread Ayurvedic literature. These factors, however, have been changing since the 1920s. Ayurveda now has been recognized and become more integrated into mainstream Indian culture, and research and development are being supported by government funding. There is also more literature in a variety of languages and translations of works previously available only in Sanskrit. In addition, there is a small but growing body of more recent literature that outlines some theoretical and practical aspects of Ayurveda (Corcos, 1984; Dube, 1979; Frawley & Lad, 1986; Jee, 1895 / 1993; Lad, 1984; Lele, 1986; Manyam, 1990; Ranade, 1993; Ranade, Ranade, Qutab, & Deshpande, 1997; Svoboda, 1992).

The classical traditions of Charaka and Sushruta have long been esteemed as constituting the very core of all Ayurvedic knowledge and practice. They have been adapted to the varying times, prevailing trends, and exigencies of their day. Ayurveda, as presented here, will take a centrist position. The classical sources are considered the bedrock foundation of timeless, enduring truths. In the spirit of Ayurveda, however, these fundamentals have been and are now applied, in a flexible way, with adaptations to include accommodation to the current culture in which they now emerge. These adjustments, in fact, have been a skillful means of helping to usher Ayurveda into modern times while striving to preserve the qualitative heart of the authentic Ayurvedic system.

Ayurvedic knowledge is thus to be understood in both intuitive and logical terms. It may be considered an empirical science since its naturalistic methodology combines a trust in the wisdom and experience of the past with an applicability that is both artful and scientific in the widest sense. As such it becomes a living, flexible reality kept fresh by reason and by the creative use of an intuitive sensitivity. It would be imprecise to view Ayurveda as a closed or dogmatic system; rather, it is one in which judicious uncertainty mixes with contemplation, reason, and time-honored guidelines.

The term *Ayurveda* is composed of two Sanskrit words, *ayus* meaning the period of life and longevity, and *veda* meaning revealed knowledge or wisdom. Ayurveda, in many contemporary contexts, has been called "the science of life." Ayurveda, however, may also be expressed by the phrase "life wisdom," which connotes its pragmatic, judicious, diligent, and mature vision. Ayurveda always had and continues to have a strong empirical and pragmatic foundation. It is scientific in that it is an organized body of theories at times used in an explanatory fashion and at other times used propositionally to be tested through experience. Western science and rational medicine evolved based on a highly logical series of systematic observations made scientific by repeated tests of validity and reliability. This experimental method requires evidence, which, over time, proves consistently true and verifiable. Modern statistical analysis accompanies most of current Western science and medicine. This method of using evidence-based approaches even goes beyond the Western world and has become part of most contemporary and modern pursuits in those areas. Approaches, such as Ayurveda, have long histories, and while their proponents regard these approaches as having been "proven" over time they may be regarded by others as less or even unscientific. The scientific view, so to speak, if considered from the larger historical perspective of the development of medicine, must become less exclusionary. Eastern medical perspectives that have been outside of the mainstream medicine of the West because of geographical, cultural, and language barriers need examination. Current trends not only permit but also demand such openmindedness. The increasing global awareness that characterizes the beginning of the third millennium mandates lifting the constraining perspectives of the past. Ayurveda, as presented here, may not fall under the aegis of being "scientific" in the accepted Western sense. Ayurveda, whether or not it may ever lend itself to more "scientific" methodologies, may accurately be seen as a parallel, alternative, or complementary system standing on its own merits and deserving serious consideration for historical, if not pragmatic, reasons.

DARSHANAS

In the complex history of ideological systems, India has been prolific and fruitful (Coward & Raja, 1990; Dasgupta, 1975; Jha, 1984; Kadar, 1996; Muller, 1899; Potter, 1994; Yukteswar, 1894/1990). Traditionally, most Indian or Hindu philosophical and religious schools of thought (*darshanas*) orient themselves around the authority of the Vedas although some remain apparently more independent. Those systems that regard the Vedas as primary revelation, as axiomatic, and as their authoritative foundation are characterized as being orthodox and true to the Vedas. They are termed *astika*. In contrast, those groups originating in the Indian culture, such as, for example, Buddhism, Jainism, and Charvaka, that either deny or reject the primary authority of the Vedas are characterized as unorthodox as well as nontheistic. They are collectively referred to as the *nastika* schools. While both perspectives have influenced Ayurveda to varying degrees, the *astika darshana* systems remain preeminent.

The term *darshana* is usually translated as *philosophical system, worldview,* or *religious system*. This vision of reality refers to the content of a particular *darshana*. In fact, *darshana* was originally used to denote the direct, intuitive experience of "seeing" reality as it existed both on the apparent level and at the essential, subtle, and root level. The *darshanas* were traditionally communicated in an oral fashion from teacher (*guru*) to student or disciple (*chela*). When written down, the body of a *darshana* was considered to fall into one of two categories: *sruti* or *smriti*. *Sruti* was understood to be the "heard," oral teachings of the *rishis* or sages who "saw" their content. This meaning applied whether or not these ideas were transcribed in written form. The Vedas and the Upanishads are thought to be in the *sruti* class of scriptural documents. *Smriti* (tradition), whether in written form or not, was understood to be the large body of commentary written about the more primary *sruti* (revelation). The classic epics, *Bhagavad Gita,* and the *Ramayana,* the narrative literature of the Puranic period (c. A.D. 320–520), and later Vedanta formulations (c. A.D. 9th–12th century) may be considered works of *smriti.*

Each of the six major *astika darshana* schools attempts to explain reality by using a particular and differing perspective.

1. *Sankhya* is the *darshana* that provides a more nontheistic creation sequence, which is used to outline the evolution and manifestation of spirit into matter. This system is one of the oldest Vedic *darshanas,* and forms the foundation of the Ayurvedic worldview. It is based on the primacy of consciousness as the integral ground that pervades and maintains the entire universe. Its originator is considered to be Kapila, one of the ancient seers mentioned in the *Rig-Veda.* The figure of Kapila remains anonymous and no details of his life have been recorded. The main *Sankhya* text is the *Sankhya Karika,* a commentary in verse on *Sankhya* by Ishvara Krishna written about A.D. 200.

2. *Yoga* is the *darshana* developed by the Indian sage Patanjali. It contains a more theistic base and describes an eightfold path characterized by introspection, meditation, self-discipline, and aspects of renunciation and asceticism. These procedures aim toward the gradual liberation of the human spirit from its bondage to the material world, a process of release referred to as *Kaivalya,* and a state of being called *Samadhi* (enlightenment).

3. *Nyaya darshana,* the method of thorough investigation, is a monotheistic system that describes a logical approach to apprehending the world by using reason. *Nyaya* has been called *Tarkavidya,* the science of debate, and *Vadavidya,* the science of discussion. This epistemological method is one of logical realism and considers that it is possible to arrive at a valid knowledge of an objective reality, a world that is independent of the mind. Perception, inference, comparison, and testimony were its epistemological axioms. *Nyaya* contains a natural theology; its

worldview admits both factual material properties, i.e., atoms and immaterial substances such as the consciousness of man. The founder of *Nyaya* has several appellations: Gotama, Gautama, Santananda, and Aksapada. He presumably lived between the sixth and third centuries B.C. and authored an important Hindu law book, *Dharma Shastra,* whose 12 volumes discuss creation, transmigration, liberation, and dharmic mandates. He also composed the *Nyaya Sutras,* a fundamental *Nyaya* text.

4. *Vaisheshika darshana* describes a complex categorical system of classification of material substances, their action potentials, and their properties or attributes. This is called *Dravyaguna Shastra.* Included in these formulations were theories of atoms and primal Elements. The primal Elements are termed in Sanskrit, the *Mahabhutanis* or *Mahabhutas.* These "great" Elements are five in number (Ether, Air, Fire, Water, and Earth) and constitute the primordial material building blocks or principles of all substances. They play a pivotal role in every aspect of Ayurvedic theory and practice. *Vaisheshika* employs a system of pluralistic realism that is used extensively in Ayurveda in its development of a materia medica, the delineation of the mechanisms by which herbal substances affect the body's functioning, and their effects on the bodily *doshas,* the physiological principles that regulate the body's homeostasis. Ayurveda has incorporated this detailed analytic system into the fabric of almost all its theoretical principles and its diagnostic assessment techniques. This system was founded in the second century B.C. by the sage Ulaka, better known by his surname, Kanada. He is said to have been the abbot of a school for priests, and to have written the first version of the *Vaisheshika Sutra* in which he introduced a theory of the atom.

5. *Purva Mimamsa darshana* contains elements of the Vedic-based philosophies with an extremely strong emphasis on the discipline, religious ritual, service, and right action that are considered significant Vedic mandates (*vidhi*). *Mimamsa* means exegesis or inquiry and this school was especially attentive to the language of the Vedas and their precise meanings. It espoused the philosophical tenets of realism and pluralism and eschewed what it regarded as idealistic conceptualizations. The founder of this school was Jaimini about whom little is known.

6. *Uttara Mimamsa* or *Advaita Vedanta* is a more spiritually oriented system that emphasizes the essential spiritual base of all reality (*Brahman*), human misperception (*advaita* and *maya*), and ways that the individual and the Ultimate may become reestablished in their already eternal axiomatic unity. The highly renowned sage, Sankara (A.D. 788–820) established a *darshana* that tends to be nontheistic and monistic. It has the philosophical features of an absolute idealism and has been one of the most influential schools of Hindu thought. It espouses a "consciousness model" as its irreducible axiomatic base.

The three *Nastika Darshanas* are Buddhism, Jainism founded by Vardhamana/Mahavira (sixth to fifth century B.C.), and Lokayata of Charvaka (c. 600 B.C.). Of these three, Buddhism has played an outstanding role in the development of Ayurveda. Its influence is inestimable. The work of the great sage and Ayurvedic physician, Nagarjuna, continues to exert a profound influence in modern times especially in the field of Ayurvedic iatrochemistry and mineral-based therapeutic preparations.

EPISTEMOLOGY

The epistemological perspective that Ayurveda uses comes chiefly from the Vedic observational system termed the *Nyaya darshana* and includes a method of means or proofs for knowledge. The instrument or organ of subjective epistemological experience is termed *Antahkarana*. This process comprises sensation, perception, concept formation, and interpretation. The four cognitive faculties subsumed within *Antahkarana* are the following.

1. *Manas*. This is the broad Sanskrit term encompassing the mind as it experiences sensations and perceptions, registers their data input, and then begins the process of identification and conceptualization.
2. *Chitta*. This is usually considered part of the function of *Manas* that specifically acts as a disseminator or transmitter from *Manas* to the higher cognitive functions within *Ahamkara* and *Buddhi*.

3. *Ahamkara*. This aspect of mind is considered the differentiated ego or individuality of the person, the self. *Ahamkara* is the specific identity of an individual or a substance. In the individual, a major function of *Ahamkara* is to evaluate the goodness or badness of an identified experience. *Ahamkara* acts as the stamp of individuality that organizes perceptions with the distinctive interpretative character unique to that individual. The function of *Ahamkara* as the self-identity provides that individual with the experience of relative constancy, sameness, and adaptable continuity over time.
4. *Buddhi*. This is the most refined aspect of the epistemological process, and is termed intellect or intelligence. Its specific connotation suggests that its functioning is most discerning with an intrinsically valid and accurate capacity to interpret experience. The *Buddhi* function decides whether one will act or refrain from acting. This is the aspect of mind closest to the innate wisdom (*prajna)* emanating from pure consciousness. The functions of *Buddhi* transcend mere physiological cognition.

Four techniques for knowing (*Pramanas*) are described:

1. *Pratyaksha,* direct sensory perception. This involves the straight contact of the five senses (sight, hearing, smell, touch, and taste) with their objects of perception. In Ayurveda, *Pratyaksha* is regarded as the preeminent mode of experiencing the material world. It is firsthand experiential sensory evidence. It is considered the premier epistemological method for ascertaining a true perceptual understanding of reality. It is believed to be the most reliable method used to arrive at a proof, a reality-based conclusion, with the reliability of *Sabda* or textual theory considered of secondary and merely supporting value. *Pratyaksha* is understood to be the proper use of the function of *Manas,* the mind. This experience is not merely a simple act of sensory perception, but, in fact, it is the experiencing of perception by living in the five senses with a focus on the perception of sensations. Dwelling within the experience of the five senses and not on their already internalized referents in the form of concepts

and preestablished understanding is the sense that *Pratyaksha* conveys.

2. *Anumana,* inference. This involves the inductive process of initial observation and data gathering, such as assessing signs and symptoms, and then the generation of explanatory hypotheses.

3. *Sabda* or *Aptopadesha,* authoritative statement. This "testimony" includes the use of texts, documents, and theories describing relevant material. In ancient times, *Sabda* (sound, hearing) was the primary form of all learning and involved face-to-face contact with a recognized teacher. This time-honored system was referred to as *guru-sisya parampara,* the transmission of knowledge from generation to generation via an oral tradition. In addition to this more direct instruction, the actual first-hand reports of patients and their families are used to gather further medical and lifestyle history.

4. *Upamana,* analogy. This *Pramana* or technique for attaining correct knowledge is the method of using abductive reasoning and relying on the best available explanation to be the truest at that time for that situation.

AYURVEDIC WORLDVIEW

The broad base, the Weltanschauung or worldview, that Ayurveda espouses is essentially unitary and dynamic. The whole of reality is conceived as an integrated coherence with actively interdependent aspects. There is no part of the totality of existence that is functionally separate or disconnected from any other. The dynamic aspect of this is fueled by the constant interaction, in biological life, amongst the three *doshas, Vata, Pitta,* and *Kapha,* all of which are the three fundamental regulatory principles of the body's physiological functioning. Since these *doshas* have an almost axiomatic role in Ayurveda, synonyms for them are generally not used. *Vata* connotes movement; *Pitta* connotes transformation; and *Kapha* suggests consolidation and inertia. The interplay between these principles modulates the interactions of the *gurvadi gunas* or 10 pairs of opposite qualities that characterize all perceptible substances. An almost infinite variety of presentations thus becomes possible.

The place of man in greater nature is reflected in the notion of "microcosm within macrocosm" or *pinda-brahmanda*. This suggests an intimate correspondence, if not virtual identity, between the life of the individual and the life of the world around. This cosmic homology is a central tenet of the Vedas. Man, in this view, is regarded as a miniature of nature, a world within a world. This connotes that everything existing in the universe is in some way encapsulated within man. Some implications of this include the intimate effect that nature or the environment has on man; for example, the influence of seasonal changes; and the presumption that all aspects of the outer world are, in some way, represented within the individual. Each individual is understood to be a unity composed of body, mind, and consciousness. The Vedic, spiritual base with an emphasis on consciousness is an important part of the Ayurvedic perspective. Ayurveda, per se, positions the physical body and its functioning in both its balanced and unbalanced states as one major focal point. Ayurveda's focus, in fact, is on the complete individual–physical body, mind, and consciousness. Since ordinary attention is most concentrated on the more material aspects of experience, Ayurveda uses the natural focal point of the body as a vehicle to begin its approach toward understanding and treating the total person.

SANSKRIT

Another important consideration in outlining the scope of Ayurveda is an appreciation of the original language, Vedic Sanskrit, in which the ancient texts were composed. Sanskrit is one of the oldest known languages. Legend states that the ancient seers or *rishis* of India developed this system of sound, speech, language, and writing during deep contemplative states. Sanskrit words were believed to reflect and contain the energetic bases of the objects or experiences to which they referred. The oldest Veda, the *Rig-Veda,* was, in fact, a text of chants or hymns.

These *mantras*, as they are called, were believed to have a magical power able to effect change. Sanskrit is held to be a sacred language by Hindus, and Ayurveda follows this view. The conceptualizations to which many Sanskrit terms refer are difficult to adequately translate and are used in their orignal form. For historical and scholarly purposes, we will provide English approximations of some relevant Sanskrit terms (Apte, 1993; Bender, 1967; Fischer-Schreiber, Ehrhard, & Friedrichs, 1994; Staal, 1963). Of note is the language called *Pali*. It is a derivative of Sanskrit and thought to be the Indian dialect used by the Buddha. Buddhists consider *Pali* a revered language and many Buddhist scriptural texts are written in this dialect, as well as in Sanskrit.

VEDIC STANDARDS AND VALUES

There are four basic life goals (*purushartha*) or prime values for each individual according to the Vedas. The fundamental importance of these and their relevance for Ayurveda is supported by Charaka's mention of them in his description of the origins of Ayurveda. They are:

1. *Dharma*, destiny, purpose, duty, obligations, immanent cosmic lawfulness, justice, and righteousness in life. This goal broadly refers to career, vocation, and the conduct of one's life; in addition, it may be understood as one's life's work or mission.
2. *Artha*, possessions. This refers to the necessary material accumulations that one acquires in order to live with a reasonable degree of comfort. Charaka specifically denotes *artha* as being the possessions or objects of the five senses.
3. *Kama*, pleasure. This is the experience that derives from the capacity of desire and relates to the natural propensity of attraction to objects that, it is felt, will satisfy needs, reduce tension, and yield wholesome pleasure or enjoyment.
4. *Moksha*, liberation. This is the central and primary goal under which the other three are subsumed. *Moksha* refers to the gradual process of becoming freed from inordinate desires

through the exercise of proper discrimination of a hierarchy of values that regards self-actualization and expanded consciousness as ultimate goals to be actively pursued. *Moksha,* in the Vedic sense, means to regain consciousness of the unity of the individual spirit (*atman*) and the universal Absolute (*Brahman*).

PRINCIPLES OF TREATMENT

The term *upasaya* refers to Ayurveda's two basic principles of treatment:

1. *Samanya,* "like increases like." This principle relates to the interconnectedness of all aspects of the world, as previously mentioned. Factors, substances, qualities, or attributes of a specific type exert similar effects on the object to which they are applied. This holds for both positive and for negative influences. The phenomenon of "like attracts like" is also included in this principle. Homologous constituents in foods and herbs, when consumed, are attracted to and assimilated into their corresponding sites in the body's tissues.
2. *Vishesha,* "opposites balance and so cure each other." This principle relates to the idea of balance and imbalance. The idea of restoring balance through applying qualities opposite to those manifesting in the imbalanced condition is especially related to more material phenomena such as the gross aspects of the physical body, foods, and herbs. Cooling substances like milk or coconut oil, for example, when ingested or applied to the body diminish excess heat and thus treat conditions such as hyperacidity or skin irritation.

UNIVERSAL DESCRIPTIVE QUALITIES IN NATURE: *SAGUNAS*

Ayurveda has constructed a detailed classification system relying heavily on the perceptual five senses; these descriptors are used to identify and characterize the essential properties of virtually all substances. These descriptive attributes or qualities are called the *gurvadi gunas* and consist of 10 pairs of opposites. The term *guna* has the connotation of being a physical and chemical property of a substance. All created realities in nature have qualities and attributes, and so are considered to be *saguna* or describable. It is customary to describe the gunic attributes of a substance using English terms.

1. *shita/ushna,* cold / hot
2. *snigdha/ruksha,* wet or oily / dry
3. *guru/laghu,* heavy / light
4. *sthula/sukshma,* gross / subtle
5. *sandra/drava,* dense / liquid
6. *sthira/chala,* stable / mobile
7. *manda/tikshna,* dull / sharp
8. *mridu/kathina,* soft / hard
9. *slakshna/khara,* smooth / rough
10. *picchila/sishada,* sticky / clear

The importance and utility of this conceptualization comprises a large part of the Ayurvedic methodology. Foods and herbal substances are understood in this way. The functioning of the body and the interplay of the *doshas* are described in these terms. In addition, virtually any perceptible data can be described using this system. This becomes useful since each attribute carries with it a distinctive set of characteristics, which are both explanatory and suggestive of potential therapeutic actions. These gunic properties have been associated with material substances and also with psychological processes. The close and, perhaps, unfamiliar juxtaposition of physical and material attributes with emotional states, for instance, is a regular part of traditional thinking in Ayurveda. In addition to the customary denotation of each term, Ayurveda adds further meanings, some of which describe states or conditions, and some of which describe functioning, processes, or trends. Ayurveda places great stress on the value of human perception. The five senses (hearing, touch, sight, taste, and smell) are the basis for contact with the world, data gathering, and for the process of inductive reasoning. The exquisite development of sensory perception is a prerequisite, therefore, for the process of correct conceptualization and deductive reasoning. This again attests to the empirical and experiential method of a naturalistic science rather than a more a priori theoretical operational style. In addition, there is a high regard for the significance of the material world rather than a deemphasis of it. This valuation of the physical body and the physical world should not be underestimated; it was and continues to be among the dominant values of the Vedas and the ancient Vedic view of the meaning of life.

The following is a brief outline of some important aspects associated with the 10 pairs of opposite qualities; they are most often referred to using their English designations:

Cold is said to induce contraction, numbness, fear, and insensitivity. The action of stopping flow by cooling (*stambhana*) is thus produced. A reasonable degree of cold, such as is experienced in the cooler seasons, is considered to encourage health by maintaining tissue viability. Cold is an essential aspect of the potency or energy (*virya*) of foods and herbs. *Kapha* and *Vata dosha* are increased; *Pitta dosha* is decreased (KV+, P−). This notation system, applicable to each different attribute, indicates that, when the designated attribute is present, then each of the three *doshas* is either relatively increased (+) or relatively decreased (−). In this particular case, *Kapha* and *Vata* are increased (+), and *Pitta* is decreased (−).

Hot increases digestion and the metabolic fire (*Agni*). It induces expansion, perspiration, inflammation, and anger. Excessive heat as experienced in the hotter seasons is not considered beneficial to health. Heat, like cold, is a prime quality of the potency (*virya*) of food and herbs. (KV−, P+, *Agni*+). In addition to the decrease in *Kapha* and *Vata,* there is an increase in *Pitta* and in *Agni,* the digestive fire.

Wet or *oily* is often termed *unctuous*. It induces lubrication, smoothness, moisture (*kledana*). The emotions of love and compassion are associated with this quality. (KP+, V−).

Dry is related to lack of moisture, absorption (*shoshana*), constipation, and anxiety. The quality of dryness is perceived chiefly through sight. (KP−, V+).

Heavy is a quality most associated with weight, fullness, and difficulty in digestion. Heavy foods contribute to building body tissues (*brimhana*). (K+, VP−).

Light is associated with less gross materials, easy digestion, and the reduction of body tissues (*langhana*). (K−, VP+, *Agni*+).

Gross has the action of covering (*samvarana*) and is associated with an increase in material structure, coarseness, crudeness, obstruction, and obesity. (K+, VP−).

Subtle denotes more immateriality, a pervading action (*vivarana*), the ability to rapidly enter very small spaces, and the capacity to increase emotional states. (VP+, K−).

Dense is considered to promote stability, strength, and cohesiveness. Its main action is solidifying (*prasadana*). (K+, VP−).

Liquid or *flowing* has a dissolving or liquefying action (*vilodana*). The quality of compassion is associated with the idea of flowing. (KP+, V−).

Stable or *static* creates support and firmness. Stable substances are enduring and strengthening to the body. The chief action is that of stabilization (*dharana*). Stable is associated with the emotional experience of faith. (K+, VP−, *Agni*−).

Mobile promotes movement and restlessness. Its action is stimulating (*prerana*). Mobile when steady (*sara*) is associated with *Pitta*; when erratic (*chala*), mobile is associated with *Vata*. (VP+, K−).

Dull creates a blunt quality, is sluggish, marked by slow action, and produces relaxation. It may help to pacify body elements (*shamana*). Dull is associated with mild, tissue maintaining food substances such as milk and ghee. (K+, VP−).

Sharp penetrates with an immediate action on the body associated with purification (*shodhana*) and an increase in the digestive process. (K−, VP+).

Soft has a loosening action (*shlathana*) and the tendency to remove hardness from the tissues of the body. This oily, loosening action creates softness, delicacy, relaxation, tenderness, love, and care. (KP+, V−).

Hard increases strength, rigidity, and has a hardening action (*dridhikarana*). It is related to selfishness. (KV+, P−).

Smooth connotes moisture and lubrication, and has a healing action (*ropana*). (KP+, V−).

Rough is understood by the sense of touch and has characteristics of dry texture, cracks, fissures and a scraping away action (*lekhana*). (V+, KP−).

Sticky or *cloudy* is associated with lack of perceptive capacity and with an adhering action (*lepana*). (K+, VP−).

Clear is related to spreading and diversification and has a cleansing action (*kshalana*). (VP+, K−).

SANKHYA MODEL OF CREATION

The Ayurvedic model of creation is derived from the Vedic system called *Sankhya*. This is a narrative sequence of enumeration that outlines the evolution of the cosmos from the immaterial realm to the material, manifest dimension. There are 24 prime cosmic principles (*tattvas*) that emerge out of a single, unified base. This model holds that the universe and humans share a common origin; that the individual is a microcosmic unit reflecting the larger macrocosmic universe; and that foundational, primal reality is a single immaterial essence out of which all material forms emerge. Although the 24 prime cosmic principles have an apparently logical, sequential development, they occur simultaneously and so may be coparallel in operation.

AVYAKTA

Pure existence, in its unmanifest state, is called *Avyakta*. Its absolutely transcendental being makes it indescribable and ineffable although the ancient Vedics acknowledged its reality with the Sanskrit terms: *satyam, ritam,* and *brihat*. *Satyam* implies the essential truth and reality of existence; *ritam,* the deep structure of the universe, connotes a substantive internal and lawful order that is self-perpetuating and self-correcting; and *brihat* refers to the vast and enormous breadth of its being, an infinite eternalness. The two chief components of *Avyakta* are *Purusha* and *Prakriti*; they constitute noumenal reality.

PURUSHA

Purusha is the Sanskrit term for the primal immaterial matrix out of which all else emerges. This single and absolute reality is understood to be identical with pure consciousness. *Purusha* may be considered the "World Ground" behind and at the heart of the entire universe. It is the primordially uncaused, substantival totality of the real, however it is understood. *Purusha* is one, pure, eternal, and changeless. It remains in a state of eternal activation. It is the primordial consciousness that grounds all else and all appearances. *Purusha* is regarded as the only being that is not material, and, as well, the only being that is the only truly conscious entity. In effect, *Purusha* may be considered the only being that is purely spirit and thus absolutely immaterial. *Purusha* has been called the "Seer" and the "Observer." It is not regarded, however, as having any resemblance to the concept of "mind"; rather it exists as a field of choiceless, passive awareness. It is associated with the idea of male energy and, although it is outside of creation, it is considered the ground or matrix of creation. *Purusha* is unmanifest; it has no material correlate; it is completely incorporeal and unlimited. From an ontological point of view, the nature of *Purusha* is virtually without descriptive qualities; that is, it is closest to the concept of *nirguna* (having no attributes or qualities). *Purusha,* as pristine consciousness, is regarded as the core of all existence, manifest and unmanifest. This consciousness paradigm is considered to mirror the spiritual basis of all reality.

PRAKRITI

When the primal immaterial matrix, the *Purusha,* spontaneously "moves," that is, experiences the primal emotional state of desire or the rudimentary condition of need, so to speak, then, at that moment, the first material energy, *Prakriti,* comes into being. Details of this are considered unknowable, and it is inferred that this mysterious point of movement initiates creation in a manner roughly akin to the Western conception of a "big bang" launching the origin of the universe. *Prakriti,* thus, can be thought of as emerging out of a field of zero point energy. This spontaneous synchronicity, the emergence of auspiciousness (*subha, mangala*), is regarded as the "Divine Mother" and the "Will of God." *Prakriti,* per se, is unmanifest and constitutes "Ur-Matter" or primordial nature. This primal matter or first substance is a kind of undeveloped energetic matter, also called *Pradhana*. *Prakriti* is unconscious yet dynamic and is the material that very gradually evolves into all forms of the manifest created world (*pravritti*). *Prakriti* is the first creation, and as such, is the first reality that contains qualities, attributes, or properties (*saguna*) capable of description. *Prakriti* contains the potential out of which boundaries and limitations may emerge. An ancient Vedic *sutra* (aphoristic verse) reflects *Prakriti's* creative intent: "I am One, I wish to become many." This is related to the Sanskrit idea of *abhasa* and *abhasana,* the process of the one transforming into the many.

MAHA GUNAS

The three axiomatic *Maha gunas* (great attributes) that are inherent in *Prakriti* are *Sattva, Rajas,* and *Tamas*. These *gunas* may be thought of as highly rarefied potentials that impart direction and create a unique character to that which they imbue. The term *guna* in Sanskrit means that which binds, a fundamental force promoting coherence. The *Maha gunas* are considered sacred and their subtle, yet profound actions are revered. The *gurvadi gunas,* in contrast, are considered coarser and are commonly used to describe features of material substances in everyday use. The character that the *Maha gunas,* considered "omnisubstances," impart denotes the degree of subtleness, purity, and the innate trend toward potential consciousness raising that a substance contains.

Sattva is the purest, most immaterial, and spiritual attribute within the manifest world. It is characterized by degrees of consciousness, intelligence, lightness, purity (*shuddha*), clarity, peace, harmony, equilibrium, and optimal balance. The simple word *goodness* aptly connotes its meaning. *Sattva* denotes the highest level of purity that is unadulterated and thus wholesome. *Rajas* is characterized by dynamic movement, kinetic energy, turbulence, agitation, change, and transformation. *Tamas* is the quality of inertia, solidity, dullness, darkness, veiling, coarseness, grossness, and materiality.

The *Maha gunas* are inextricably bound up with *Prakriti* and remain the most essential and overridingly influential aspects of all of her developed forms. The binding forces and trends at the heart of all creation events emanate from the *Maha gunas*. When in perfect balance, the *Maha gunas* create a more spiritual or immaterial state in the created object. The usual condition of creation, however, is imbalance of these *gunas*. To the corresponding extent that *Sattva* is less prominent, a more material, corporeal, gross, or imperfect state of being exists. Out of these primordial *Maha gunas* come the more materially perceptible *gurvadi gunas* that are the intrinsic properties of substances in the world recognizable by the five senses.

MAHAT

At this juncture in the creation sequence, the previous aspects that were noumenal in nature first begin to become manifest and their phenomenality, more material, defining, and specific properties begin to be consolidated. These cosmic principles that make up nature or *Prakriti,* according to the *Sankya* system, continue to be human centered and so have what may be seen as an anthropomorphic orientation.

The first manifestation, which is considered to have some developed primordial material substance, is called *Mahat* (cosmic intelligence). This is understood to be the innate intelligence within all aspects of the universe. This innate intelligence is made up of laws and regulatory principles (*ritam* and *dharma*) that determine the course of evolution. *Mahat* is the transitional area between noumenal and phenomenal reality; it has been called the "Divine Mind." Within the individual, *Mahat* is termed the *Buddhi,* the reliable capacity to discriminate truth from falsehood, right from wrong, reality from delusion and illusion. Intelligence, therefore, in this view, comes into being prior to the grosser forms of matter that only later evolve into existence.

Another important aspect of *Mahat* is its containment of what are called the *Pancha Tattvas* or five root causes that eventually create the five sense organs (*jnanendriyas*), the five motor organs (*karmendriyas*), the five *tanmatras* or subtle energies behind the five elements, and the five great gross Elements (*Pancha Mahabhutanis*). *Mahat* is regarded as the first organization out of *Prakriti* that is a nodal intelligence having coherence and direction, and being capable of imparting the rudimentary template of form. This is the genesis of the *Maha gunas: Sattva, Rajas,* and *Tamas*. The *Pancha Tattvas* within *Mahat,* therefore, are understood to be the spiritualized, seed precursors and the spiritual etiological stimuli behind and at the heart of the entire created world.

AHAMKARA

The next step in the developmental process of *Prakriti* is a giant leap and is what eventually becomes most characteristically individualized in human experience. It is called *Ahamkara*. This is the point at which unity differentiates and splits into individuality. The English word closest to this concept would be *ego*. It implies a separate and distinct delineation of self from all else, as well as a subjective and unique experiential identity characterized by feelings of separation, isolation, and difference. *Ahamkara* becomes the ego container that makes one thing unique, different, and separate from all else. For human beings, *Ahamkara* becomes the experience of a personal sense of self. It is limited self-awareness. This quality is chiefly applied to human life but is also an aspect of other sentient life, such as exists in the plant and animal world, and imparts that entity's essential identity that remains constant but which is flexible, changeable, and adaptable via modifications over time.

Through the vehicle of *Ahamkara,* both the five *Tattvas,* and the three *Maha gunas* begin to dynamically build the manifest universe. Up to this point, the quality of all created being has been *karana* or virtually spiritual in its entirety. It is also termed *causal, seed, magnetic,* or *soul*. The rest of the creation process now becomes more "incarnated" or material. There is a trend downward, so to speak, into grosser, more concrete, and tangible manifestations of reality.

BIRTH OF THE *DOSHAS*

As *Sattva* interacts with *Rajas* and *Tamas*, the kinetic energy of *Rajas* precipitates out what is to be the vital, energetic essence that pervades all biological life, *Prana*. This *Prana* or life force is identical with what in traditional Chinese medicine is called *Qi*. Out of this *Prana* comes the first bioenergetic *dosha, Vata*. Out of *Vata* come the other two *doshas, Pitta* and *Kapha*. This broad level of reality, having both spiritual as well as more grossly material qualities, is metaphysically termed *sukshma*, the subtle, energetic, or vital level. The older literature has referred to this as the "astral" sphere.

The concept of the *doshas* forms a bedrock group of axioms in Ayurveda. They have traditionally been called "humors" which implies the historically archaic conceptualization found in ancient Greek, Roman, and Unani Tibb medical texts. The idea of *dosha*, as a biological and energetic substance, originates in the work of Charaka and then Sushruta, the ancient authors of the original and still fundamental Ayurvedic texts. The Sanskrit word *dosha* literally means spoiling, fault, or darkener. This refers to the *dosha*'s inherent capacity to become vitiated or agitated and disruptive of the current status quo. This apparent disruptive action is, in fact, a positive homeostatic mechanism aimed at regulating the health of the body. The connotation of being a disrupter suggests the dynamic action that is inherent in the functioning of the *doshas*. The concept of *dosha* contains two most fundamental ideas: (1) its being a bioenergetic substance and (2) its acting as a bioenergetic regulatory physiological force, process, or principle. The nature of *dosha* is that of a force that resides on the borderline between matter and energy. Since the *doshas* do have material substance, they are, in part, composed of varying amounts of what are called the five great gross Elements (*Pancha Mahabhutanis*) that are the five elemental building blocks of all matter. They are Ether, Air, Fire, Water, and Earth. These "primary pentads," as they are sometimes called, are the very first precipitations of material substance, and compose the elemental building blocks and internal regulatory principles that make up the *doshas*.

Doshas, in general, however, exert their effects in a more functional way in the human body. They are the basic organizing principles that regulate and maintain physical and psychological homeostasis. In effect, they are the intermediaries between the outside world (foods, diet, seasons, daily routine, lifestyle) and the tissues, systems, and functioning of the body. These homeostatic regulators act as protective barriers guarding the health and integrity of the body both mental and physical. The connotation of the *doshas* as faults refers to the fact that the *doshas,* as protective intermediaries, can be disrupted, imbalanced, and temporarily impaired. This process has been traditionally referred to as "vitiation," a customary and standardized term denoting a pathological state of a *dosha.*

Vata

Vata has been called the biological air humor. *Vata* means wind and suggests movement. Its main characteristic is that of propulsion. *Vata* is responsible for all motion in the body from the cellular to the tissue and musculoskeletal level; for the coordination of the senses; for the equilibrium of the tissues; for the acuity of the senses; and for respiration. The central and peripheral nervous system is under the control of *Vata*. Since it has a primary leadership role, *Vata* has been referred to as the "king *dosha.*" In fact, one might also view the nature of *Vata* as being a "servant *dosha*" since it is the only *dosha* that serves the other two by acting as their vehicle and carrier within the paths of their operation. It transports them and itself to peripheral sites in the body. Like *Pitta* and *Kapha dosha, Vata* has a base in the sattvic *Maha guna* (purity), but, unlike the other two *doshas,* it has a significantly larger complement of the rajasic *Maha guna* (turbulence). This rajasic aspect is the basis for *Vata*'s kinetic action. In terms of the 10 pairs of descriptive *gunas, Vata* has the following qualities: cold, dry, light, subtle, mobile, sharp, hard, rough, and clear. *Vata* is composed of the Ether (*Akasha*) Element and the Air (*Vayu*) Element.

Pitta

Pitta is known as the biological fire humor. Its etymological derivation is associated with digestion, heating, and transformation. *Pitta*'s chief action is that of digestion or transformation from the cellular, tissue, and organ level to the psychological, mental, and emotional spheres. Conversion and thermogenesis are prime activities of *Pitta*. The fundamental Ayurvedic concept of *Agni*, or digestive fire, is inextricably tied into the activity of *Pitta dosha*. The key attributes of *Pitta* are hot, slightly oily, light, subtle, mobile, sharp, soft, smooth, clear, and flowing. *Pitta* is composed of the Fire (*Tejas* or *Agni*) Element and the Water (*Ap, Apas,* or *Jala*) Element. *Pitta* has a strong sattvic base and also contains a significant measure of the rajasic *Maha guna*.

Kapha

Kapha has been called the biological water humor. Its chief characteristic is that of cohesion and binding. The word *Kapha* means phlegm and suggests the quality of connectedness. *Kapha* maintains the stability of the bodily tissues and imparts a quality of protection, which is related to its tendency toward denseness, containment, and materiality. The qualities of *Kapha* include cold, wet, heavy, gross, stable, dull, soft, smooth, cloudy, and dense. *Kapha* is composed of the Water Element (*Ap, Apas, Jala*) and the Earth (*Prithvi*) Element. *Kapha* has a base in the sattvic *Maha guna* but contains a significant measure of the tamasic *Maha guna* (inertia).

PANCHA TANMATRAS

As we continue our analytic descent in describing the sequence of the origination of the world around us, we come to the beginnings of the five *Tanmatras*. They are sometimes referred to as the "Subtle Essences." They are the subtle energies that are behind and that generate the manifestations of the next phase in evolution: (1) the Five Great Gross or Material Elements; and (2) the five sense organs of perception.

The five *Tanmatras* (underlying subtle energies), their corollary sense organ, and primary Element correspondences are:

1. *Shabda Tanmatra*: the energy that generates sound via the ears; its chief primary Element is Ether.
2. *Sparsha Tanmatra*: the energy that generates touch via the skin; its chief primary Element is Air.
3. *Rupa Tanmatra*: the energy that generates sight via the eyes; its chief primary Element is Fire.
4. *Rasa Tanmatra*: the energy that generates taste via the tongue; its chief primary Element is Water.
5. *Gandha Tanmatra*: the energy that generates smell via the nose; its chief primary Element is Earth.

FIVE GREAT GROSS ELEMENTS: *PANCHA MAHABHUTANI*

The five great gross Elements or Primordial Pentads are known as the *Pancha Mahabhutani(s)* or *Pancha Mahabhuta(s)*. They exist on the most material level (*sthula*). These five Elements, the primary pentads, are conceptualized as the first and most elemental substances that compose matter; and they function as principles of density. In addition, they also carry a strong metaphorical connotation that implies their being a representation of physiological functioning when considered from the viewpoint of biological life. Varying mixtures of one or more of these Elements compose and are the material "stuff" of all manifest reality, including the mind. Mind in Ayurveda has a distinctly material connotation. This broad conceptual perspective holds that immaterial consciousness manifests materially first in the form of the five great Elements. These Elements constitute degrees of density of matter. They represent stages in the manifestation of consciousness as progressive levels of increasing density and materiality (Table 2.1).

The five Elements are:

TABLE 2.1
***Pancha Mahabhutanis*, the Five Great Gross Elements.**

Akasha, Ether
Vayu, Air
Tejas, Fire
Jala, Water
Prithvi, Earth

1. *Akasha,* Ether. This is the first Element to precipitate out of the five *Tanmatras*. It is, in fact, transitional, in that it is the only Element that is completely subtle with virtually no material quality. Ether is characterized by the qualities of nonresistance, space, and receptivity. Its attributes include being subtle, soft, and light.
2. *Vayu* or *Marat,* Air. Out of Ether comes the Element Air. Movement and direction characterize it, and its attributes include being light, dry, subtle, cold, and dispersive.
3. *Tejas,* Fire. As Air continues to move and cause friction, the Element of Fire emerges. Fire has the manifested qualities of light, appearance, and energy. Its qualities include being hot, penetrating, subtle, light, and dry.
4. *Jala,* Water. Ancient texts say that Fire causes the densification of consciousness that becomes Water, which has the quality of flowing and allows for a potential cohesion of life. Its qualities include its being fluid, soft, and sticky.
5. *Prithvi,* Earth. As Water coagulates, it transforms into Earth, a mass that is dense, stable, and solid. Its qualities include its being gross, stable, heavy, and hard.

PANCHA JNANENDRIYANI

The next phase in the cycle of creation is that of the emergence of the five sense organs of perception called the *Pancha Jnanendriyani*. The critical importance of these cognitive sense organs, the resting place of the senses, in Ayurveda cannot be overstated. These sensory faculties make possible direct contact with the outside material world. This connotes the importance of the idea of the necessary and valuable experience of contact with the sensory world. The sense of touch, i.e., contact and connection, is uniquely intrinsic to every other sense modality. The sense organs flow more out of their anlagen in the five *Tanmatras*. In addition, because of their potential benefit for further human development, they are more imbued with the sattvic *Maha guna*. As mentioned above, the five sense organs are: ears (*shrotra*), skin (*tvak*), eyes (*chakshu*), tongue (*jihva*), and nose (*grahana*). Their respective objects are: *shabda* (sound), *sparsha* (touch), *rupa* (form), *rasa* (taste), and *gandha* (scent or aroma). Varying amounts and combinations of the five great gross Elements make up each of these objects of the senses.

PANCHA KARMENDRIYANI

On the same conceptual level as the five sense organs, there exist correspondences with the five organs of action, the *Pancha Karmendriyani*. Their more material nature is associated with their emergence from the five great Elements and their more action-oriented functioning is the result of their greater content of the rajasic *Maha guna*.

An outline of the action organs and their correspondences to function, sense organ, and Element are: (1) Mouth (*vak*): speech, ear, and Ether; (2) Hands (*pani*): holding, skin, and Air; (3) Feet (*pad*): walking, eyes, and Fire; (4) Urogenital (*upastha*): procreation, tongue, and Water; (5) Anus (*payu*): excretion, nose, and Earth.

MANAS

The *Sankhya* enumeration now describes the distinctively human faculty, mind or *Manas*. While most English translations use the term *mind* to indicate the nature of *Manas*, *Manas* also refers to the general process of thinking, mentation, and sequential experience. *Manas* is understood to be "fed" by impressions resulting from the five sensory organs of perception and the five motor organs of action. These faculties are termed *indriyas*. *Manas* can be conceived of as the "sixth sense" whose objects and contacts act within the intrapsychic or internal mental arena. It has been called "lord" of the five cognitive senses. *Manas* is a unifying and formulating principle that includes the integrated functioning of sensory perception, conceptualization, and some degree of conation or volitional activity.

Manas thus connects the individual both to the outside world and, as well, to what is interior, having a degree of apperception, so to speak. *Manas,* in addition, may be roughly equated with the Western psychological concept of ego or personality with particular emphasis on affects and all the mechanisms of defense such as denial, repression, splitting, etc. The defense mechanism of intellectualization is especially highlighted. These actions of *Manas* along with the normative "spoiling" functions of the *doshas* constitute the ground that makes for human proneness to corruption, fraudulence, and inauthenticity in both body and mind. The allied concept of the mind's intrinsic cognitive fault, *Prajna-aparada,* will be discussed at length in chapter 6.

As each individual person is, to varying degrees, "his own person," he or she thus manifests a personal *Ahamkara*. Once born into the world, all experience imprints itself on the individual and thereby modifies and shapes individual identity. This conditioning (*samskara*), so to speak, of *Ahamkara,* is facilitated by *Manas*. Attachment to a personal sense of self is a chief function of *Manas*. Inherent in the idea of the connectedness that *Manas* mediates between the senses and its attraction–attachment to the outside world is the phenomenon of the experience of desire (*mara, raga, trishna, iccha, abhinivesha*). *Manas* can be thought of as a functional key, the ticket of admission, to the experiential world. It constitutes the point of contact between inner man and the world. Desire, operative within the functioning of *Manas,* in all its expressions is held to be among the most fundamental driving forces in human nature. The phenomenon of desire denotes both the unconscious and the conscious craving for satisfaction, gratification, and fulfillment of subjectively experienced wishes. The perpetual drive toward wish fulfillment, a pathognomonic feature of man's mind in Eastern traditions, acts both as a motor and as an organizing set of mental impulses that strive to repetitively achieve previously experienced satisfactions. The problem of "glamour," the uncanny excitement and pull (*upadana*) that the material world has on the mind, is intimately tied in with the functioning of *Manas*. This phenomenon is termed *Vishaya-Shakti*, the power of the world of the senses. The function of *Manas*, by its inherent nature, tends to create a linkage, dependence, or bondage (*bandha*) to the sense objects of the material world. The regulation of desire, then, becomes a central theme in the Ayurvedic system of health, well-being, and self-development. This follows from the premise that Ayurveda seeks to address the needs of the physical dimensions of life, the body and the mind. In the course of achieving and maintaining a healthy physical balance, further harmony is induced on what are considered more spiritual and consciousness enhancing dimensions. In Ayurveda, the fact of the body's being the physical base of consciousness, its material dimension, is never lost sight of.

The distinctions, then, between different aspects of psychic functioning are as follows. The Sanskrit term *Manas* denotes the broad idea of mind as it experiences desire, needs, and cravings elicited through sensory experience, and possessing the wish for pleasure and gratification. *Chitta* is a term roughly synonymous with *Manas* but containing the idea of having relay capabilities providing connections to other mental functions. The Sanskrit term *Chitam* denotes the general concept of mind as a seat of consciousness with dimensions that are conscious, unconscious, and transcendently conscious or superconscious. *Buddhi* is the inherently intelligent aspect of mind that is most sattvic (pure, conscious, balanced) and has the power to correctly discriminate that which is good and conducive to growth, maturation, and development (*satyma*) from that which is unwholesome (*asatyma*).

HEALTH, BALANCE, PURITY, AND WHOLESOMENESS

Lastly, the Ayurvedic concept of health is based on the idea of achieving dynamic balance. When the *doshas* are in balance, health ensues. The state of the *doshas* determines the state of all other aspects of the individual—digestion, elimination, tissue integrity, energy level, mental and emotional stability, and optimal overall functioning, to name just a few. Striving for balance is an ongoing task and is fostered and supported by continuing efforts toward maintaining purity (*shuddha*) on all levels of one's being. Optimal *Agni*, the transformational fire that pervades the entire individual and which brings about maximal nutrition in body, mind, and spirit, accompanies the optimal balance and functioning of the *doshas*. Purity, health, and wholesomeness (*satyma*), therefore, are achieved through prescribed dietary practices, daily and seasonal routines, and healthy lifestyle activities that include material and spiritual dimensions. In addition to the care of the body, care of the mind and spirit includes meditative practices and other self-inquiry pursuits.

Maintenance of the health of the body is not only an end in itself, but also a prerequisite to further development on more refined levels. This includes the psychological, the subtle-energetic, and the spiritual. This idea rests on several propositions fundamental to Ayurveda. The first is that of the primacy of consciousness, and its primordial ontological position. Today, even outside of Ayurveda, the examination of the qualitatively unique significance of consciousness and its critical role in human culture is a generally recognized fact (Block, Flanagan, & Guzeldere, 1997; Cairns-Smith, 1996; Hameroff, Kaszniak, & Scott, 1996; Neumann, 1954; Solso, 1999). In the Ayurvedic worldview, as consciousness participates in the evolutionary process, it gradually manifests in forms that are denser and have increasingly denser material attributes, like the physical body. The individual's purpose in life, therefore, is to become aware of the immanence of consciousness at the core of physicality, and to facilitate and enhance its manifestation process. Accordingly, man has the directive to experience his material reality to its fullest accompanied by this realization. The second proposition then entails the goal of maintaining the optimal health of the body in order to provide an adequate amount of time for a higher quality of life to be achieved. In the Buddhist tradition, the term *kushala* or wholesomeness connotes those activities of daily living that have high degrees of purity and an absence of inordinate avarice, greed, aggression, hate, and cognitive confusion. Pursuit of wholesomeness, in this sense, is considered to be of great value since it is believed to purify one's *karma,* that is, to contribute to freeing one from the fetters of unresolved conflicts and bondage stemming from the past. The ultimate aim of this is the achievement of the prime Vedic goal, *moksha,* that is, liberation into ever higher states of consciousness.

CHAPTER 3

ANATOMY

THE PHYSICAL BODY AND ITS COMPONENTS

Ayurvedic anatomy (*Sharira Rachana*) is a description of the morphological constituents of the individual and an enumeration of the integrated material structures and principles through which the various physiological processes occur. The physical body, in fact, is viewed as the material expression of man's essential core, that is, of consciousness. As was described in the preceding outline of the *Sankhya* creation sequence, the immaterial aspects of reality, particularly the reality of consciousness, are given primacy in terms of origin, value, and significance. The physical body (*sthula sharira*), however, remains the material ballast of man's consciousness, and is regarded as the platform upon which all endeavors for well-being must begin.

The basic components of the body are the humors (*doshas*), the tissues (*dhatus*), the secondary tissues (*upadhatus*), the tissue membranes (*dhara kalas*), the channels of circulation (*srotas*), the waste products or refuse (*malas*), and the organs. Each of these will be discussed here. The *srotas,* which have more of a physiological function, will be discussed in a later chapter.

DOSHAS AND SUBDOSHAS

The concept of the *doshas* is a major focal point in Ayurveda. Ayurvedic evaluation is based on an assessment of the state and interaction of the *doshas* in the body. Health and disease is reflected in the condition of the *doshas*. Treatment, as well, is based on efforts to balance vitiations in the doshic system. As described previously, there are three *doshas*: *Vata* is the principle of propulsion; *Pitta* is the principle of transformation; and *Kapha* is the principle of consolidation (Table 3.1).

TABLE 3.1
***Doshas* and their Subdoshas**

Vata

1. Prana Vata
2. Udana Vata
3. Samana Vata
4. Apana Vata
5. Vyana Vata

Pitta

1. Pachaka Pitta
2. Ranjaka Pitta
3. Sadhaka Pitta
4. Alochaka Pitta
5. Bhrajaka Pitta

Kapha

1. Kledaka Kapha
2. Avalambaka Kapha
3. Bodhaka Kapha
4. Tarpaka Kapha
5. Shleshaka Kapha

Vata

Vata has been described as having characteristics of both a bioenergetic substance and a regulatory principle. *Vata* is the *dosha* closest to having the properties of immateriality, that is, acting as a more amorphous energetic entity. Although *Vata* has no form, its presence can be likened to that of the energetic transmissions that travel through the nervous system, or to the motion that accompanies breathing. From an anatomical perspective, the chief seat or "home" of *Vata* is in the large intestine or colon. This specificity refers to the fact that the primary site of accumulation of *Vata,* especially in disease, occurs in the colon. In addition, *Vata*'s influence is also concentrated in such sites as the hips, thighs, ears, trachea, bones, brain, and skin. Each of the three *doshas* is subdivided into five components. The subdoshas of *Vata* are termed *Prana, Udana, Samana, Apana,* and *Vyana*. Vata is considered the lead *dosha* since only this *dosha* has the primary function of propulsion that applies to it and its role in moving and propelling both *Pitta* and *Kapha*. Some have referred to *Vata* as the first equal among the three equally primary *doshas* (Figure 3.1).

Prana Vata pervades the brain, heart, and lungs. Each of the five senses, especially those of hearing and touch, is imbued with the activity of *Prana Vata*. *Prana* means forward or primary air. It governs and supports respiration, heart rate, the vegetative and the sensory functions. It has been associated with the actions of inhalation, swallowing, sneezing, spitting, and belching. It is the main and directing form of all the other *Vata* subdoshas. The subtle roots of *Prana,* as the life force, are considered the connecting links to consciousness, and cultivation of *Prana* is held in high regard. *Prana* is absorbed instantly via the air inhaled into the lungs, and in a delayed fashion via the absorption of food in the colon.

Udana Vata is concentrated in the throat, chest, lungs, navel, and sinuses. *Udana* means upwardly moving air. It governs exhalation, speech, coughing, vomiting, and belching. Along with speech expression and communication, *Udana* governs memory, remembrance, and will or volition.

Samana Vata perfuses the whole alimentary tract, especially the small intestine. It regulates peristalsis. *Samana* means the equalizing or balancing air. It balances the energy of the body and is very closely tied to assimilation, in general, and specifically to the digestive process. This encompasses the assimilation of food in the gastrointestinal tract, air into the lungs, and sensory experience into the mind. In addition, *Samana Vata* is the predominant *Vata* in the internal organs including liver, spleen, pancreas, stomach, and upper part of the large intestine. It also

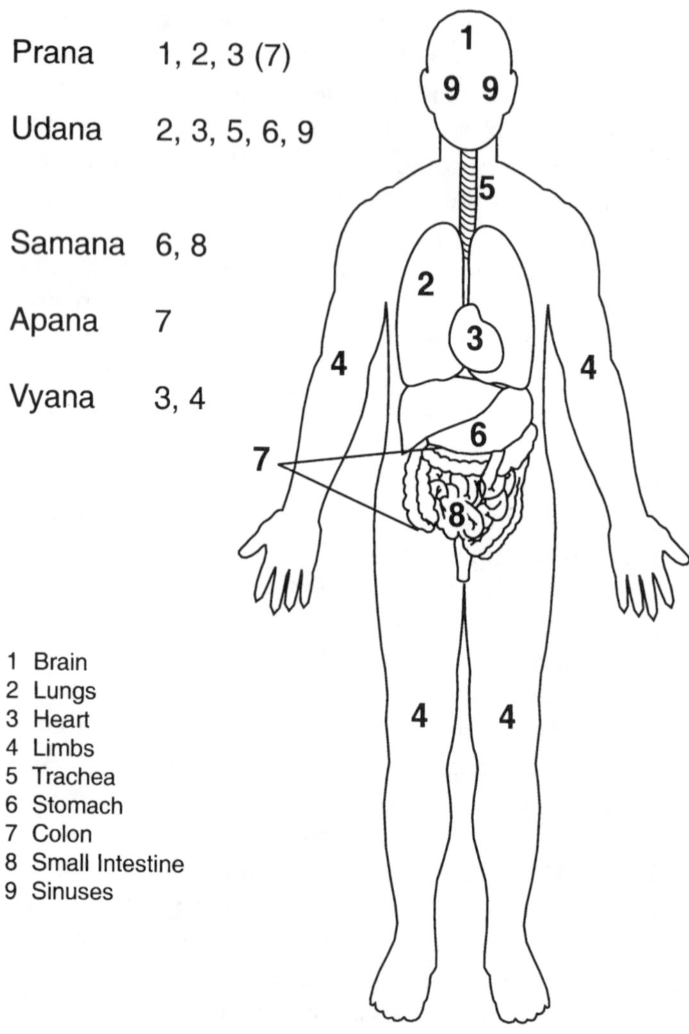

Figure 3.1. The five subdoshas of *Vata*: Primary anatomical sites.

contributes to movement in the blood circulatory system and the nervous system.

Apana Vata is centered in the colon and controls the other *Vata* subdoshas. *Apana* means downward moving air. In addition to absorbing *Prana* from food in the colon, *Apana* is the chief *dosha* directing all elimination. This includes excretion of feces and urine, and includes menstruation, parturition, and sexual discharge. The state of *Apana Vata* is critical in Ayurvedic evaluation since it reflects, to a significant extent, the overall health or disease of the individual.

Vyana Vata is contained in heart, blood vessels, skin, bones, muscles, and nerves. *Vyana* means diffusive or pervasive air. The chief actions of *Vyana Vata* are the circulation of blood from the heart to the periphery, the movements of the musculoskeletal system, and the innervation of the sensory organs. The processes of blinking and yawning have been associated with it.

Pitta

Pitta is the *dosha* that drives change and transformative processes. Its chief site is in the small intestine. This is the anatomical place in which it will accumulate when it becomes vitiated and excessive. *Pitta* is also found in the liver, spleen, stomach, skin, eyes, heart, and parts of the brain; it is also present in sweat, sebaceous oil, blood and, to a small degree, in lymph. Bodily warmth and heat, essential to life, emanates from *Pitta*. *Pitta's* five subdoshas are *Pachaka, Ranjaka, Sadhaka, Alochaka,* and *Bhrajaka* (Figure 3.2).

Pachaka Pitta, the *Pitta* of digestion, is located mainly in the small intestine and lower stomach, and is contained in hydrochloric acid, enzymes, bile, and hormones. It is the main *Pitta* involved in the second or sour phase of primary digestion (*avasthapaka*) and its actions assist in regulating body temperature and fueling the strength of circulation. Its functioning is tied into the operation of *Agni,* the fundamental digestive fire of the body. This also puts it close to the actions of another digestion-related subdosha, *Samana Vata. Pachaka Pitta* controls and supports all other *Pitta* subdoshas.

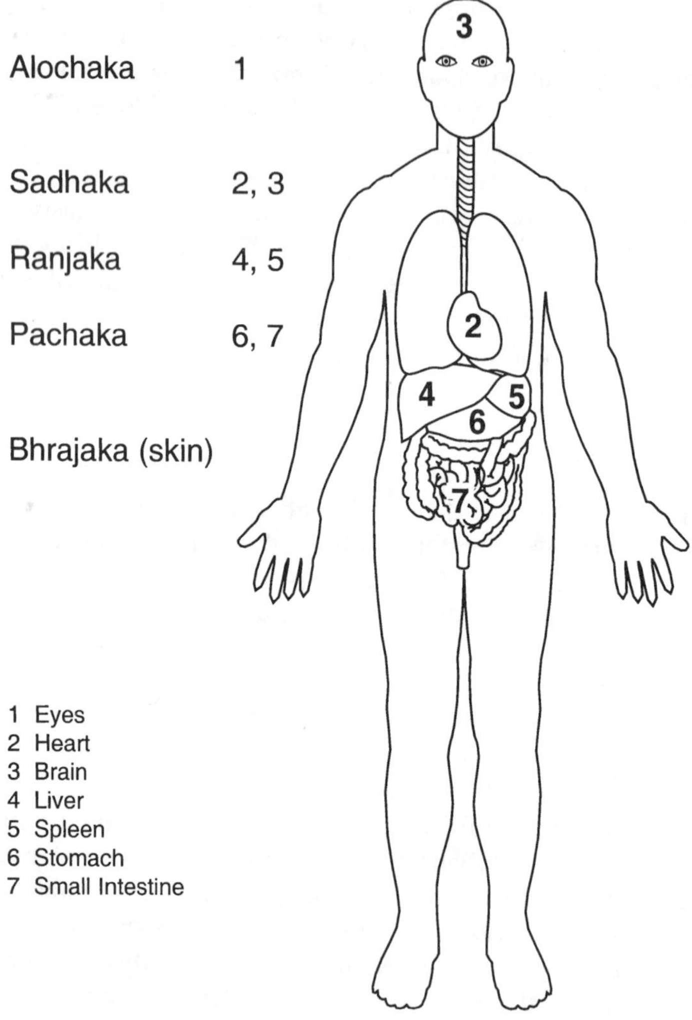

Figure 3.2. The five subdoshas of *Pitta*: Primary anatomical sites.

Ranjaka Pitta, the *Pitta* that gives color, resides chiefly in the liver, spleen, small intestine, stomach, blood, bile, and stool. This *Pitta* is mainly associated with secondary digestion which is referred to as "tissue metabolism" whose site is in the liver. This *Pitta* contributes to erythropoiesis, the formation of red blood cells.

Sadhaka Pitta is located in the heart and brain. *Sadhaka* means accomplishment, realization, and discernment. It functions through the nervous system and sensory organs to produce clear thinking, intelligence, recognition, comprehension, memory, courage, and contentment. Cultivation of this *Pitta* can propel the individual toward realization of the four goals of life according to the Vedas: *dharma, artha, kama,* and *moksha. Sadhaka Pitta* energizes the acuity of the *Buddhi* aspect of mind. On the other hand, many forms of desire and lust are associated with *Sadhaka's* penetrating power.

Alochaka Pitta is the *Pitta* of the eyes and governs visual perception. In addition, *Alochaka Pitta* contributes to the functioning of all the other sensory organs to some degree.

Bhrajaka Pitta is located in the skin, the sweat, and the sebaceous oils. It is the *Pitta* fire that governs luster of the complexion. It is also related to the temperature of the skin.

Kapha

The word *Kapha* means "water flourishing." *Kapha dosha* is the *dosha* of body fluids such as plasma, mucus, phlegm, cerebrospinal fluid, and synovial fluids. *Kapha* is the most material, dense, gross, and coarse of the three *doshas*. *Kapha* engenders form, has a tendency toward solidity of form, and imparts protection from inordinate heat and wear and tear of everyday functioning. The five subdoshas of *Kapha* are *Kledaka, Avalambaka, Bodhaka, Tarpaka,* and *Shleshaka* (Figure 3.3).

Kledaka Kapha is located in the stomach. It means the form of water that moistens or humidifies. Its primary action is to liquefy food in the alkaline or sweet phase of the first stage of digestion. In addition, it protects the stomach lining from damage by excess *Pachaka Pitta* and *Agni*, the digestive fire.

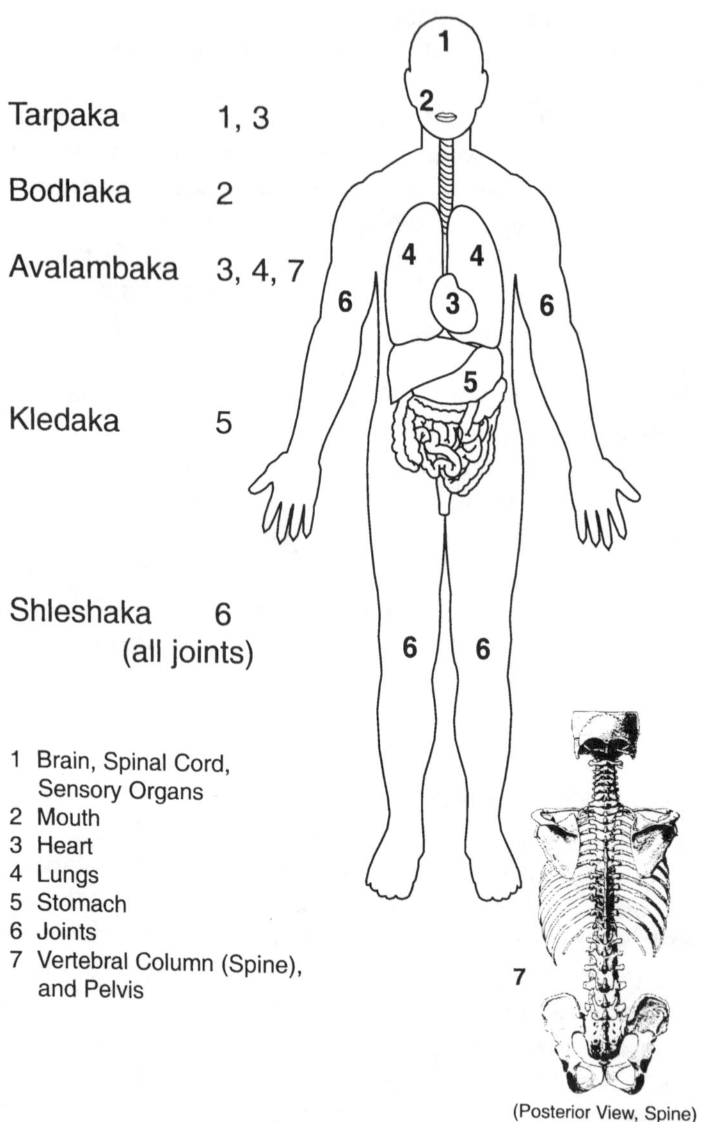

Figure 3.3. The five subdoshas of *Kapha*: Primary anatomical sites.

Avalambaka Kapha is located in the heart, lungs, spine, and pelvic girdle. It is the form of water that gives support. In the chest, it provides lubrication for the heart and lungs. It is a central, supportive component for the stability of the vertebral column. *Avalambaka Kapha* is the central *Kapha* and controls all other *Kapha* subdoshas. Its fundamental significance lies in the fact that it is the force behind the first and primary body tissue (*dhatu*), the plasma (*rasa*). In Ayurveda, the plasma is considered the matrix tissue out of which all other tissues are formed. *Avalambaka Kapha* is considered the material medium associated with psychological attachment and detachment, love and depression.

Bodhaka Kapha is located in the tongue, mouth, and in the saliva. It means that form of water that gives perception. This *Kapha* subdosha has also been called *Rasana Kapha. Bodhaka* is the subdosha related to taste. The Sanskrit word for *taste* is identical to that for *plasma,* the first bodily tissue to be formed and upon which all other tissues develop. Plasma and taste are both termed *rasa* because of their functional association in Ayurvedic physiology. Taste, a critical faculty in the Ayurvedic scheme, is that sensory guide that not only is a screen to determine the nature and wholesomeness of a substance, but also becomes therapeutic when herbs of differing tastes are used to balance excess *doshas*. Healthy plasma is reflected in a state of healthy, balanced *doshas,* and both are a consequence of the ingestion of the proper tastes being consumed. In this sense, the specific Ayurvedic concept of "taste" is distinct from the meaning of the common word *flavor,* which is nonspecific, general, and more inclusive.

Tarpaka Kapha is located in the brain, cerebrospinal fluid, heart, and in the sinuses. It means that form of water that gives contentment (*tripti*). *Tarpaka Kapha* has also been called *Snehana Kapha. Tarpaka* is associated with emotional stability and peace of mind. Some Ayurvedic sources consider it to be the physical source and container of consciousness. It has been called the *dosha* that nourishes the sense organs of perception (*jnanendriyas*). In conjunction with *Prana Vata,* its balanced functioning assuages anxiety and insomnia.

Shleshaka Kapha is the synovial fluid within the body's joints and articular surfaces. It means lubrication and stickiness.

SUBTLE OR ENERGETIC ROOTS OF THE *DOSHAS*: *PRANA*, *TEJAS*, AND *OJAS*

The concept of the *doshas*, as has been discussed, is one of the fundamental working frames of reference in Ayurveda. The *doshas* are bioenergetic both in substance and in functioning. They tend to be more material in nature, and so reside in and make up part of the physical body (*sharira sthula*) and work through physiological processes. As the whole of the Ayurvedic worldview is one of dynamic, multidimensional integrated functioning, an elaboration of the deeper aspects of the *doshas* reveals their subtle counterparts that reside on the vital or energetic level. The subtle roots of *Vata*, *Pitta*, and *Kapha* are *Prana*, *Tejas*, and *Ojas*, respectively.

Prana

Prana is the subtle root of the coarser, more material subdosha *Prana Vata*. *Prana* is considered the life force, and has been called *Qi* in Chinese traditional medicine. *Prana* is subjectively experienced as the will to live. The significance of *Prana* lies in the fact that it exerts an integrative drive toward confluence of all aspects of the individual on all levels. As the life force, *Prana* is indwelling in the individual but does need to be replenished on a daily basis. The rudiments of what transforms into the vital Pranic substance come into the body through air and through food. *Pranayama* is the system of intentional and conscious breath regulation to facilitate the absorption of *Prana* into the lungs and bloodstream. Eating fresh foods, especially of reasonably high quality, and taking specific herbal substances, also increases the body's concentration of *Prana*.

Tejas

Tejas is the subtle root of the coarser, more material subdosha *Sadhaka Pitta*. *Tejas* is considered the flame of life, and its functioning of interactive transformation makes it closely allied to *Agni,* the overall digestive fire. In traditional Chinese medicine, the concept of *Yang* is most closely related to the concept of *Tejas*. In Ayurveda, *Tejas* functions chiefly as the transformative force of penetrating intelligence and discrimination. As such, it is closely connected to the *Buddhi* aspect of mind. The quality of *Tejas,* as well, is related to the quality of personal self-discipline and determination. Its integrative action effects a penetration that reaches all material and subtle aspects of the individual so that they may mutually influence each other.

Ojas

Ojas is the body's vital essence that is manifest by and contained in the *Tarpaka Kapha* subdosha. *Ojas* means vigor and strength. It can be considered a substance that is transitional between the physical and the energetic spheres in the body. Some Ayurvedic writers have described *Ojas* as being the nexus substance between consciousness and matter. Unlike *Prana* and *Tejas, Ojas* has more physical or material reality. Some Ayurvedic texts regard *Ojas* as a highly rarefied tissue substance. In traditional Chinese medicine, the Ayurvedic concept of *Ojas* is most closely identified with that of *Yin* and with that of *Jing*. Enduring immunity, enduring memory, and the quality of peace of mind or contentment (*tripti*) have been considered functions of *Ojas*. *Ojas* is regarded as the primary energy reserve of the body. It is the ultimate product of nutrition, digestion, and metabolism. Ayurveda regards the subtle dimension of the heart (heart *chakra*) to contain several drops of the best *Ojas* (*Para Ojas*). The major portion, however, termed *Apara Ojas,* is distributed throughout the rest of the body.

THE SEVEN BODILY TISSUES: *SAPTA DHATUS*

The universe is considered to be constructed with seven planes of existence (*sapta lokas*). The body, in similar fashion, is understood as being composed of seven basic tissue elements (*sapta dhatus*). The Sanskrit word *dhatu* means that which enters into the formation of the body as a whole in order to hold and support. These seven bodily constituents are composed of all five Elements, but, as in the case of the *doshas*, only one or two Elements predominate in each tissue. The entire body is composed of the seven tissues, and these tissues sustain the organized material structure of the individual. Although both are considered physical substances, the *doshas* take on more of a functional and regulatory role while the tissues provide the integrated physical matrix within which the *doshas* operate. There is a definite sequence of tissue production in the body. This spans a range from most gross with the largest mass and least compact quality toward most subtle, having less mass, and a greater degree of compactness (*samhana*). The first tissue and "most gross or material" substance is called the plasma (*rasa*); next is blood (*rakta*), then muscle (*mamsa*), fat (*meda*), bone (*asthi*), marrow and nerve (*majja*), and lastly, reproductive (*shukra*). In Ayurvedic tradition, the *Ojas*, being considered the supremely vital, life-sustaining essence, has been sometimes called the "eighth tissue."

Plasma

Plasma (*rasa*) is chiefly composed of the Water Element. It constitutes the chyle, lymph, serum, or plasma matrix that bathes all the other tissues. The Ayurvedic concept of *rasa* is, in fact, much broader than the Western medical definition of plasma. *Rasa* is the total water content of the body, which amounts to about 55% of body weight and is the most abundant constituent of the body. The Western definition of plasma, on the other hand, is restricted to denote only the intravascular water that contains electrolytes and clotting factors. In the circulatory vessels, this intravascular plasma is the medium in which red blood cells, white blood cells, and platelets are contained. Extracellular water occupies two main body spaces: (1) the intravascular spaces

(25%) comprised of the blood and lymph in their circulatory vessels; and (2) the interstitial spaces (75%) comprised of the areas around cells, blood vessels, and all other tissues. In Ayurveda, however, the concept of *rasa* includes the total body water contained in both the intracelluar and the extracellular body compartments. *Rasa,* therefore, denotes the massive pool of life sustaining substances permeating all the *dhatus* (tissues) in the entire body.

The intimate association between the Ayurvedic concept of taste (*rasa*) and the plasma tissue (*rasa*) has profound implications, and this is implied since the Sanskrit term for both is identical. The nutritive and therapeutic value of an ingested substance, i.e., food and herbs, is determined by the combination of tastes that it contains and evokes. These materials, when properly digested, become the first bodily tissue, the *rasa,* which acts as the foundation for all further nutrition and tissue production. *Rasa* is considered the first point at which digested food transforms into the human *Ahamkara* with an individualized, specifically human identity. Plasma has been called the "sap" of the body and, as such, its function is to provide nutrition and nourishment for every other component of the body. Generation and maintenance of the physical body has its repeated beginnings and further development at the juncture at which *rasa* is made. All vital nutrients are in solution and are distributed via the plasma. The Sanskrit word *prinana* is used to describe the action of the plasma. *Prinana* connotes fulfillment, fullness, hydration, pleasure, and the expectation of more to come. In the Ayurvedic sense, the *prinana* aspect of *rasa* results from the pleasure that is considered to be the subjective experience resulting from the circulation of *rasa.* The predominant *dosha* contained in plasma is *Kapha,* particularly the *Avalambaka Kapha.*

Although all seven tissues are of vital importance, the developmentally first, the plasma, which launches the evolution of the tissue formation chain, is one of the most important tissues that determines the health or disease of the body. The plasma, therefore, is the basic nutritive matrix for the entire bodily substance, and, as well, is the basic matrix out of which all other tissues develop.

Each tissue is considered to have a "membrane" that may be both a material covering and have functional and physiological significance. These tissue membranes or *dhara kalas* are nutritive membranes within and around the tissue and around that tissue's specific channel or circulatory system. These membranes not only seal and protect the tissue substance but also filter out wastes in addition to facilitating the absorption and diffusion of nutrients that feed the tissue. Each tissue membrane is the main site of that tissue's particular digestive fire (*dhatu Agni*). The membrane structures associated with the plasma are called *sleshmadhara kala*. *Sleshma* is an ancient synonym for *Kapha* and connotes the virtual identity of plasma and *Kapha*. It is believed that the synovial membranes around joints are specifically related to these plasma-*Kapha* membranes.

Blood

Blood (*rakta*) is chiefly composed of the Fire and Water Elements. It is the particulate matter in the circulatory system, especially the erythrocytes or red blood cells. Its unique status, which makes it essential to life, has prompted Ayurvedic tradition to virtually regard it as the fourth *dosha*. A chief function of blood is to carry oxygen and to oxygenate all the other tissues. In addition to this, blood is considered to vitalize and to invigorate; in this respect, its functioning is referred to as *jivana* (invigoration). The Sanskrit term for blood, *rakta,* means that which is colored red. This connotes blood's warmth and stimulating capacities. Along with its ability to carry oxygen, blood is the gross fluid that holds and carries the *Prana* or vital energy. Blood is closely identified with *Ranjaka Pitta*. Blood thus functions to oxygenate the tissues, to contribute to the circulation of *Prana,* and to induce a sense of invigoration, ardor, and passion.

The membranes associated with the blood are called *pittadhara kala*. This connotes the intimate connection between the blood and *Pitta,* its origin. In Ayurveda, the *pittadhara kala* are considered to have their anatomical sites not only in the endothelial lining of the blood vessels but also in the membranes of the gastrointestinal tract, especially the small intestine. The *dhatu-Agni* (tissue fire of digestion) of *Ranjaka Pitta*, situated in the liver, is the primary site of the secondary metabolism or general tissue metabolism, which occurs after the primary digestive process in the stomach and the small intestine.

Muscle

Muscle (*mamsa*) is composed chiefly of the Earth Element with some additional Water and Fire Elements. Muscle imparts strength and has the function of plastering or binding (*lepana*). The connotation of the root of the term *mamsa* suggests the function of holding firm. The membrane that holds muscle tissue is called *mamsadhara kala*. It is usually associated with the anatomical structures of the deep fascia.

Fat

Fat (*meda*) is composed chiefly of the Water Element. Its function is that of lubrication (*snehana*). The term for fat, *meda*, denotes that which is oily. This tissue has been traditionally associated with the melodious functioning of the voice, and also with the emotion of loving affection. The membranes that are associated with fat are called *medodhara kala*. These are anatomically associated with the greater and lesser omentum, sheaths of fascia in the abdominal area anterior to the lower parts of the stomach and to the transverse colon.

Bone

Bone (*asthi*) is composed of the two Elements: Earth and Air. Its function is support (*dharana*). The Sanskrit term for bone, *asthi*, means to stand or to endure. Bone is the physical container of the *Vata dosha*, particularly *Vyana Vata* and *Apana Vata*. The membranes that contain and nourish it are called the *purishadhara kala*. These periosteal membranes, according to Ayurveda, are intimately associated with the mucous membranes of the large intestine or colon. Any *Vata* imbalance, normally having its seat of perturbation centered in the colon, therefore, will ultimately affect the skeletal system (*asthi dhatu*) in some manner. Although this association appears unusual, it is a traditional Ayurvedic concept and has great therapeutic significance, particularly demonstrated by the efficacy of therapeutic enemas used in the treatment of bone disorders.

Marrow and Nerve Tissue

Marrow and nerve (*majja*) is composed of the Water Element. In Ayurveda, the function of marrow is to produce fullness and contentment (*purana*). The meaning of marrow derives from the root *maj,* which denotes sinking. This is understood to suggest that which is sunk and encased in bone. This encompasses both bone marrow and the entire central and peripheral nervous system. All the *Vatas* circulate through the marrow and nervous system or *majja*. The membrane that holds the marrow and nerves is referred to as *majjadhara kala* (marrow and nerve nutritive membrane).

Reproductive Tissue

Reproductive tissue (*shukra*), both male and female, is composed of the Water Element. It is considered to be the essence derived from all the tissues, especially the marrow and nerve tissues. Its multiple functions include producing progeny, giving strength, producing energy, and fostering stamina. The Sanskrit word for reproductive tissue, *shukra,* means seed and luminous. It also refers to the planet Venus. The membranes that hold reproductive fluids are called *shukradhara kala* (reproductive tissue nutritive membranes).

SEQUENCE OF TISSUE DEVELOPMENT AND NUTRITION

In the developmental origin and production of the bodily tissues, the first tissue to be formed is believed to be the plasma.

When food (*ahara*) is taken into the mouth, it is considered "unhomologous." In Ayurveda, this means that its individual identity (*Ahamkara*) continues to be retained. Since this is experienced by the body as foreign at first, it is not fully utilizable. In the process of digestion in the stomach and small intestine, the "raw" unhomologous material begins to be transformed into useful nutrition. At this point, this "preplasma" is called *ahara rasa,* the still unhomologous nutritive substance. Once the *ahara rasa* enters the liver and is digested by the appropriate transformative processes, it then becomes a homologous chylelike fluid and is called *rasa* proper or plasma. Through a series of ongoing and dynamic processes, this assimilable plasma is used for nutrition, and also is used for the process of transformation into the other tissues in a sequential manner. Plasma transforms into blood, blood into muscle, muscle into fat, fat into bone, bone into marrow, and marrow into semen.

This direct, transformative sequence of tissue formation (*Ksheera Dadhi*) is a dynamic process that produces ongoing stable tissue (*sthayi dhatus*), unstable tissue (*asthayi dhatu*), gross waste products (*sthula mala*), subtle waste products (*kleda*), and secondary tissues (*upadhatus*). There are two other theories of the mechanism of the transformation of one tissue into the next. The first is called *Kedara Kula* and refers to the channel irrigation method used on farms. Nutrients travel through the blood vessels to nourish and produce tissues. The second is called *Kale Kapota* and means the "land and pigeon" selectivity mechanism wherein each tissue extracts the specific nutrients it needs from the plasma so that it may grow and develop. The time sequences for tissue productions vary. Plasma is developed daily and transforms into blood in about 5 days. The full transformation of plasma into reproductive fluid is believed to occur in about 35 days.

BODILY WASTE PRODUCTS (*SHARIRA MALAS*) DERIVED FROM FOOD

The body produces three main gross waste products (*sharira malas*) from the intake of food after all digestion is completed:

urine (*mutra*), feces (*purisha*), and sweat (*sveda*). These are considered functionally important although they are ultimately the discardable end products of ingested food. Urine is derived from the intake of water and the metabolic fluid wastes. The function of the urine is considered to be the carrying away of wastewater (*kleda vahanam*). The basic portion of urine is first in the colon and then extracted into the circulation to go through the channels (*srotas*) so that *kleda* or wastes may be collected and carried away to the kidneys for excretion. Sweat is believed to be an end product derived originally from the intake of air. Its main function is considered to be the process (*kleda vidhruti*) of separating waste from nutritive material. Sweat brings *kleda* wastes to the skin, not only to dispel them, but also for the purposes of moisturizing and oiling the skin. Feces are originally derived from the food or *ahara* intake. In addition to its obvious function of ridding the body of excrement, Ayurveda highlights its dual supportive roles. Feces are considered to have a primary role called *avasthamabhana;* this refers to the function of supporting the structure and tone of the colon and the entire pelvic area. In addition, the feces are believed to support the *Agni* or digestive fire and contribute to the body's normal temperature regulation.

SECONDARY TISSUES OR *UPADHATUS*

As the primary seven tissues (*dhatus*) are produced, they also produce accessory or secondary tissues (*upadhatus*). The primary tissues maintain the functioning of the secondary and supplementary tissues. *Rasa* produces *sthanya* (breast milk) and *raja* or *artava* (menstrual fluid). *Rakta* produces *sira* (blood vessels) and *kandara* (tendons). *Mamsa* produces *vasa* (muscle fat), *tvacha* (skin), and *snayu* (ligaments). *Meda* produces omentum sheaths around fat, small tendons, and small bony joints. *Asthi* produces *danta* (teeth). *Majja* produces *dushika* (sclerotic fluid of the eyes). *Shukra* produces *Ojas,* the bodily fluids associated with immune functions.

GROSS WASTE PRODUCTS DERIVED FROM TISSUE METABOLISM (*DHATU MALAS*)

The gross waste products of the tissues (*dhatu malas*) are considered significant byproducts necessary for the health of the body. Along with the formation of these tissue gross byproducts, a small amount of subtle tissue wastes called *kleda* are also produced. *Kleda* constitutes an amorphous mixture of waste materials that have moist and evaporative properties but no other coarser correlates in the body that can be measured in appreciable amounts.

The gross tissue waste products (*dhatu malas*) resulting from their respective primary tissues (*dhatus*) are as follows. Plasma is considered to be originally derived from *Kapha*. In the process of its multiple transformative stages, plasma yields *Kapha dosha* as one of its primary tissue byproducts. Blood is believed to be originally derived from *Pitta*. Like plasma, in its multiple transformative processes, blood yields *Pitta dosha* as one of its primary tissue byproducts. Muscle is originally derived from *Kapha*. Its byproducts are called *khamalas* and are described as being the waste material found in the cavities of the body's outer surfaces: ears and nose, for example. Fat is originally derived from *Kapha* and has sweat as its major gross tissue waste product. Bone is originally derived from *Vata dosha*. Its two main gross tissue byproducts are *nakha* (nails) and *kesha* (hair).

Marrow and nerve tissues are originally derived from *Kapha* and produce the byproduct associated with the glaze or fluids of the eyes. Reproductive fluids are derived from *Kapha* and yield the byproducts of smegma and facial, axillary, and pubic hair.

Thus, after the ingestion of food, its unassimilated and post-digestive end products or gross waste products (*sharira malas*) are excreted from the body in the form of sweat, urine, and feces. Proper digestion and assimilation, therefore, ultimately produces primary tissues (*dhatus*), secondary tissues (*upadhatus*), gross tissue wastes (*dhatus malas*), very subtle tissue wastes (*kleda*), and excretory gross wastes (*sharira malas*).

GROSS ANATOMY

In Ayurveda, the detailed gross anatomy of the body is virtually similar to that described in Western medicine. The morphological and functional Ayurvedic perspective, however, is different and reflects the centrality of the *doshas* as they function in both health and disease. There are several versions of a body structure concept. The two most common are the following.

1. Head, Trunk, Branches View. The body in this view is composed of three main sections. They are (a) *shira,* the head-neck portion; (b) *kostha,* the trunk portion; and (c) *shakha,* the branches portion. The head and neck part contains both solid tissue and hollow organs. The trunk portion contains the gastrointestinal tract and most of the organs that have hollow interiors. The branches include the four limbs and are composed of the highest proportion of solid tissue such as muscle and bone.

2. Hollow Organ, Compact Tissue View. The body here also consists of three groupings. They are (a) *kostha* which includes the gastrointestinal tract, the plasma, and some hollow organs; (b) *shakha* that includes the four limbs, the blood, the muscles, and fat tissue; and (c) *marmas* or *madhyama* that includes the head-brain, the heart, the kidneys, the urinary bladder, and bone, nerve-marrow, and reproductive tissue. The *madhyama* are considered the most vital organs and tissues.

MARMA POINTS

Marma points, of which there are about 107, are significant areas on the surface of the body, which are sensitive and responsive to injury and to therapeutic pressure. The first reference to these points is found in the *Athara Veda,* an ancient Vedic text with some medical content. The later medical text, *Sushruta Samhita,* more fully expands on their locations and therapeutic use. Ayurvedic sources speculate on the possibility of these larger area *Marma* points being the progenitors of the smaller area acupuncture points used in traditional Chinese medicine. At this time, there is no material evidence to substantiate this, other than

Ayurvedic oral tradition. The antiquity of the Indian *Marma* concept is believed to extend back to a very ancient Ayurvedic medical text, the *Suchi Veda,* as yet undiscovered. *Marma* areas are defined as the anatomical site on the surface of the body where muscle, blood vessel, bones, tendons, ligaments, and joints meet. There are three major ways of classifying them: (1) by their region or area on the body; (2) by the tissues and structures of which they are predominantly composed; and (3) by the signs they produce when they are injured. By careful massage, especially with specific essential oils, *Marma* stimulation is believed to regulate the functioning of the *doshas* and the physiologic processes in the body.

The three great *Marmas* (*Mahamarmas*) are: (1) *Hridaya Marma* located over the heart area; (2) *Shira Marma* located on the head area; and (3) *Basti Marma* located over the lower abdominal area.

THE ORGANS OF THE BODY

In Ayurveda, the tissues (*dhatus*) of the body are a central focus of attention in determining health and imbalance as well as in assessing and formulating therapeutic interventions. The body's organs, important as they are, take on a secondary role. This apparent deemphasis of the organs may, in fact, be due to the Ayurvedic conception of *dosha-dhatu* (humor-tissue) structure and functioning which implicitly includes the actions of the organs although this is not made explicit in the literature or in clinical practice. Each organ, however, is correlated with its important tissue, channel, subdosha, and allied substance such as its waste product and its relevance to *Ojas,* the physical substance associated with immunity, vigor, and strength. The major organs and their correlation to the *doshas* and tissues will be outlined here.

The functioning of the gastrointestinal tract is pivotal in Ayurveda. The organs directly related to it, therefore, are of primary importance. The stomach is considered a *Kapha* organ in which the *Kledaka Kapha* is prominent. The sweet phase of primary digestion occurs here. The small intestine is the site of

Pachaka Pitta, which is intimately allied with the central *Agni* or digestive fire and is called the *Jatharagni.* The sour phase of primary digestion occurs here. The colon is the major site of *Apana Vata* and the site of the pungent phase of primary digestion.

The nature and understanding of the pancreas (*kloman*) and the spleen are important and take on a different significance from that in traditional Chinese medicine. In Ayurveda the spleen is considered a *Pitta* organ with a preponderance of *Ranjaka Pitta* similar to the liver. The spleen is understood to be involved with the production and destruction of blood components. In contrast, the pancreas is thought of as a *Kapha* organ with a preponderance of *Kledaka Kapha.* As such, it is involved in the processes of primary digestion with an emphasis on water and blood sugar regulation. For example, according to Ayurveda, the imbalances produced by diabetes and hypoglycemia, and also the clinical phenomena of nonpitting edema are related to impairments of the pancreas according to Ayurveda. In the Chinese system, however, the important concept of "damp spleen" refers more to what Ayurveda considers pancreatic disorders, although the term *pancreas* is not used in the Chinese description.

The brain is considered a central organ that houses three significant subdoshas. *Prana Vata* has its primary site in the brain. *Sadhaka Pitta* and *Tarpaka Kapha* share prominence here as well. These are vital subdoshas and have profound psychological and consciousness-related impact. The heart contains *Sadhaka Pitta, Avalambaka Kapha,* and both *Prana* and *Udana Vata.* The liver and gallbladder are imbued with *Ranjaka Pitta.* The kidneys have a predominance of *Apana Vata.* The reproductive organs of the female contain *Kapha* in the breast tissue and *Pitta* in the uterus, ovaries, and fallopian tubes. The male gonads contain *Kapha.*

Specific organs, in part, regulate the tissues and their functioning. This takes on clinical significance in disease because a diseased tissue's governing organs are believed to be also impaired and, in part, etiologically responsible for their tissue's dysfunction; therapeutic intervention, therefore, may be directed to the organs. The plasma is considered to be governed by the heart and the lungs. The heart, liver, and spleen govern the blood. The liver, spleen, and pancreas govern the muscle. The pancreas and kidneys govern fat. The colon and the kidneys govern bone. The colon is believed to be responsible for the direct nourishment of bone through the functioning of the *purishadhara kala* or colon membrane. The brain and the colon govern the marrow. The gonads and the kidney govern the reproductive fluids. This close tie of tissues with their controlling organs again demonstrates the interrelatedness of the body according to Ayurveda.

BIOPSYCHOSPIRITUAL STRUCTURAL ORGANIZATION

The Ayurvedic model of the individual is an integrative one. This conception acknowledges and describes a structural and functional interpenetration of dynamic components that include physical, psychological, and spiritual-consciousness dimensions. Ayurveda, as has been alluded to previously, emerged out of the ancient Vedas and was influenced by the work of Patanjali, the propounder of the Yoga system. The following description derives from both these traditions; its import rests in the comprehensive picture of man's multifaceted constitution that it presents.

The human body (*sharira*) may be understood as having three major aspects that range from the gross or most material level of being, through a more rarefied, subtle, or energetic level, to the most immaterial, spiritual, causal, or seed-origination sphere. Within each of these three fundamental domains, there exist differing gradations or organizational nodes called *koshas* (sheaths) in which aspects of the five Elements, the *doshas,* and the *Maha gunas* (*Sattva, Rajas, Tamas*) operate. The core at the center of these five sheaths or coverings is called *atman,* the individual spirit or consciousness. *Atman* is considered to be *Brahman,* the universal Absolute, as it exists in the individual.

The first aspect is the gross or physical body (*sharira sthula*) made up of coarse matter that has perceptible mass and is most tangible. On this level, the five great Elements (Ether, Air, Fire, Water, and Earth) predominate and create the unique physical morphology of that specific individual. The three *doshas, Vata-Pitta-Kapha* (VPK), constitute the physiological aspect of the five Elements and act as the body's functional and regulatory principles. This physical sheath is called the *Annamaya Kosha.* It has been referred to as the outermost, that is, most material, layer or dimension of the individual. This material sheath is considered relatively coarse and crude in comparison to the composition, structure, and fineness of the other dimensions that constitute the individual.

The second aspect is the subtle or energetic body (*sharira sukshma*) made up of more immaterial yet vital substances that function as the psychological, mental, and emotional spheres. It is here that the subtle forces of *Prana, Tejas,* and *Ojas* are situated. Two sheaths are organized at this level: (1) *Pranamaya Kosha,* the breath sheath: this houses the activity of *Prana* and the breath, the basic life force. This has been referred to as the "body of energy" and has been considered to have a special relation to what are called the five organs of motor action, the *karmendriyas. Pranayama* or breath exercises prevent the sensory and nervous disturbances that may occur here; (2) *Manomaya Kosha,* the emotional-mental sheath. This is the site of *Manas* (mind). This sheath has been considered to have a special relation to the organs of the five senses, the *jnanendriyas.* The practice of *mantras* and of music therapy may help to manage anxiety and thought disorders, and Yoga meditations contribute to preventing various forms of mental deterioration.

The third aspect is the spiritual or causal-seed body (*sharira karana*) constituting the most immaterial level of the human being. It is here that the quality of one's consciousness, self-realization, and awareness resides. Two sheaths are found at this most rarefied plane: (1) *Vijnanomaya Kosha,* the intelligence–wisdom–*Buddhi* sheath. *Buddhi* is the infallible intelligence that is able to discern truth from falsehood; and (2) *Anandamaya Kosha,* the bliss sheath that is considered closest to the core (*atman*) of the individual.

The Yoga concept of Patanjali regards the five sheaths as surrounding, but not touching, the primary spiritual core called *atman.* Yoga systems aim at releasing (*moksha*) the *atman* from its fetters to these sheaths and the material world. Ayurveda tends to regard the multidimensioned concept of man in a more integral way with consciousness pervading and supporting the entire unity. Cultivation of consciousness in all its manifestations, material and nonmaterial, is a Vedic precept. *Moksha* or liberation, in this sense, is regarded as freedom from the mistaken belief that man and nature, in themselves and in relation to each other, are split and divided. The Vedic concept of *moksha* denotes attaining the realization of personal wholeness within a unified field that is consciousness-based. The physical body, therefore, is more than a vessel or container of the spirit; it is the material dimension of spirit. Spirit, indivisible from matter, is an acknowledged real presence. In Ayurveda, the physical body, rather than being considered as a prison, is understood to be the medium within which consciousness unfolds. The root of the Sanskrit word *budh* means to regain consciousness. It is this consciousness of unity within apparent diversity that constitutes the Vedic view.

CONCEPT OF *CHAKRAS*

Chakras (energy wheels) are subtle energy structures or nodes organized at different sites along the spinal cord. Although they are not considered to have physical substance, they are located in the region of major nerve plexuses and exist with them but on the subtle or vital plane along a subtle channel (*nadi*) called the *sushumna*. The specific action of the *chakras* involves the concentration, organization, and regulation of the individual's vital life force, *Prana*, also called *Kundalini Shakti*. In this sense, the *chakras* are functional entities that exert an energetic and subtle physiological role. This conceptualization, used in Ayurveda, comes from the work of Patanjali and remains a significant part of the Yoga system. The Pranic life force is considered to contain the currents of consciousness. It is used in a practical way in the course of the process of meditation as a preparatory stage in which attention is withdrawn from the sensory arena and refocused on the more subtle level of the *chakras* in order to activate their specific functioning. When each *chakra* is energized in this manner, its main Pranic life force is intensified. As each of the seven *chakras* activates in this way, a progression begins from the lowest *chakra*, the *Muladhara*, up to the highest *chakra*, the *Sahasrara*. During the course of this process, the quality of one's consciousness is believed to change, clarify, intensify, and broaden.

The *Muladhara Chakra* is considered the root center and the main foundation or support for the *chakras* above. This spatial positioning refers both to physical and anatomical locations, and, as well, to the degree of subtleness and the qualitative relationship to consciousness that the *chakra* holds. This *chakra* is located in the region of the anal and perineal area and related to the sacral and coccygeal plexus. Its related *Marma* point is called *Guda*, and its primary Element is Earth.

The *Svadhisthana Chakra* is considered the sex center. It is located near the genitals and related to the hypogastric, lumbar plexus. Its related *Marma* point is *Kukundara*, and its primary Element is Water.

The *Manipura Chakra* is located near the navel and related to the solar and celiac plexuses. Its related *Marma* points are *Nabhi* and *Bruhati*, and its major Element is Fire.

The *Anahata Chakra* is located near the heart and related to the cardiac plexus. Its related *Marma* points are the *Hridaya* and the *Amsaphalaka*; its major Element is Air.

The *Vishudha Chakra* is located near the throat and the group of nerve plexuses includes the cervical, the carotid, and the pulmonary. Its related *Marma* is the *Nila Manya*, and its primary Element is Ether.

The *Ajna Chakra* is located between the eyes and related to the cavernous plexus, optic chiasma, and thalamic–hypothalamic–limbic–pituitary system. Its related *Marma* is the *Sthapani*. This *chakra* has been called the "third eye" because of its intimate connection with the meditative process and the development of refined levels of consciousness.

The *Sahasrara Chakra* has been called the crown *chakra* and occupies the area near and above the top of the head. The activation of this chakra is associated with the highest degree of the refinement of consciousness. This state of consciousness is called *Samadhi*.

CHAPTER 4

PHYSIOLOGY

Ayurvedic physiology (*sharira krija*) focuses on the functioning, processes, and mechanisms of the bodily structures. In this chapter, the systems of channels of circulation (*srotas*) that pervade the entire physical body, the concept of *Agni*, and the processes of digestion operative from the cellular through the tissue, organ, and channel system levels will be discussed.

SROTAS: THE CHANNELS OF CIRCULATION

The Ayurvedic concept of *srotas* refers to a complex interconnected system of communicating networks that perfuse all bodily substances. The term *srotas* derives from the Sanskrit root *sru* meaning "to flow." The *srotas* are considered tubular canals of circulation through which nutrients, *dhatus* (tissues), and *malas* (wastes) are produced, distributed, and eliminated. The concept of circulation in Ayurveda is not restricted only to the flow of blood and plasma throughout the body but is extended to include substances such as the *doshas*, nutrients, waste products, and even tissue elements. These *srotas* carry nutrients and waste materials both to and between the *dhatus* and the organs. *Srotas*, therefore, are involved in the formation, destruction, and conduction of *doshas, dhatus*, and *malas*. The *srotas* and the *dhara kala* (tissue membranes) are functionally and structurally related. Each *srotas* has a root organ that is considered its point of origination as well as its regulatory and controlling center. Any disturbance in an organ is reflected in a disturbance in the functioning of its *srotas*. Some Ayurvedic texts use the term *srotamsi* when referring to the plural of *srotas* although current convention is to use the term *srotas* when referring to the channel system in either the single or plural sense (Table 4.1). In a more restrictive sense, the generic concept of *srotas* may be delimited by more particular but, admittedly, loosely defined terms such as *rohini* (arteries), *nila* or *sira* (veins), *keshika* (capillaries), *gauri* (lymphatic vessels), *dhamani* (arteries, motor nerves), and *aruna* (sympathetic nerves).

TABLE 4.1
***Srotas*, the Major Channel Systems**

Pranavaha Srotas, the respiratory system
Udakavaha Srotas, the water metabolism system
Annavaha Srotas, the digestive system
Rasavaha Srotas, the plasma circulatory system
Raktavaha Srotas, the blood circulatory system
Mamsavaha Srotas, the channels of circulation for muscle tissue
Medhovaha Srotas, the channels of circulation for adipose tissue
Asthivaha Srotas, the channels of circulation for bone
Majjavaha Srotas, the channels of circulation for nerve
Shukravaha Srotas, the channels of circulation for reproductive tissue
Artavavaha Srotas, the channels of circulation of the menstrual system
Stanyavaha Srotas, the channels of circulation of the lactation system
Swedavaha Srotas, the channels of circulation for sweat
Mutravaha Srotas, the channels of circulation for urine
Purishavaha Srotas, the channels of circulation of the excretory system

Optimal flow through these channels is reflected in optimal health. Disturbed flow, causing illness, may take the following forms:

1. Excessive flow: this is usually caused by conditions that increase *Vata*.
2. Deficient flow: this is usually caused by conditions that increase *Kapha*.
3. Blocked or knotted up flow (*srotorhodha*): this is usually caused by conditions of increased *Kapha, Ama* (toxins), or waste product buildup.
4. Diverted flow out of the proper channel (*vimarga gamana*): this is caused by blockages or spasms. This is a serious condition that may damage the channel itself, and may damage the surrounding tissue. *Vimarga gamana* may produce a structural

deformity of the channel (*kervaigunya*) that may become a fundamental factor in establishing a future disease process.

5. Abnormal direction of the flow within the channel (*pratiloma*): this may result from a blockage or from a reversal of the direction of *Vata* in the channel.

There are five main classes of *srotas* containing a total of about 16 primary channels, each categorized by its particular functioning. The principal classes are: (1) intake of nutrients; (2) nutrition of tissues; (3) elimination of wastes; (4) mental and emotional functioning; and (5) female reproductive functioning. Each class has particular subdivisions, and while only 16 are primarily delineated, the actual number of channels is virtually innumerable since they pervade all areas of the entire body and consist of an intricate latticework of main and subsidiary branches.

Intake of Nutrients

Pranavaha Srotas is roughly equated with the respiratory system. The organs that constitute its origin, regulation, and control are the heart and lungs, the colon, and the brain. The functioning of this channel is intimately connected to the *Pranamaya Kosha* or breath sheath of the individual that exists on the *Pranic* or subtle level. Oxygen and *Prana* are carried in this *srotas*.

Annavaha Srotas, also called *Maha Srotas*, is equated with the functioning of the gastrointestinal tract. The areas that constitute its origin, regulation, and control are the stomach and the left side of the body. The *Maha Srotas* is one of the most important channel systems since it is the primary pathway for nutrition from the outside and its condition depends on the daily intake of proper foods and their proper assimilation. Food is carried in this channel.

Ambuvaha Srotas, also called *Udakavaha Srotas*, is the channel system that regulates the water metabolism in the body. There is no direct correspondence in the Western conception of physiology other than the functioning of organs such as the pancreas, colon, and the kidney. The origin and regulating areas of this *srotas* are the hard and soft palates in the mouth and the pancreas. Water and fluids are carried in this channel.

Nutrition of Tissues

Rasavaha Srotas is the system of vessels that carry the plasma and lymph. The areas where it originates and that regulate its functioning are the heart and the blood vessels. This is considered an especially important *srotas* since it provides the foundation for the internal nutrient pool that is the matrix for the entire body. Chyle, lymph, and plasma are carried in this channel. *Raktavaha Srotas* is the circulatory system, the system of vessels that carry blood. Its organs of origination and control are the liver and the spleen. *Mamsavaha Srotas* is the system of channels that pervade the muscles. Its origin is considered to be in the skin and the ligaments, which control it. The factors associated with muscle tissue structure and physiology are carried in this channel. *Medavaha Srotas* is the system of channels that pervade the adipose or fat tissues. Its origin and regulation is situated in the kidneys (including the adrenal glands) and the abdominal omentum. The components necessary for fat tissue are carried in this channel. *Asthivaha Srotas* is the system of channels that perfuse the osseous or bone tissues. Its origin is considered to be in adipose tissue and the pelvic bones of the hip. The components necessary for bone tissue are carried here. *Majjavaha Srotas* is the system of channels that supply the marrow and nervous system including the cerebrospinal fluid. Its origin and control sites are in the bones and in joints, and the materials related to bone marrow, cerebrospinal fluid, and nervous tissue. *Shukravaha Srotas* is the group of channels that constitute the reproductive system in the male and in the female. Its origin in the male is the testes; in the female, its origin is in the uterus and ovaries. Reproductive fluids are carried in this channel. Some texts differentiate the *Shukravaha Srotas* as being the male reproductive system in contrast to the *Artavavaha Srotas* considered the female reproductive system, and place the female *srotas* in its own class.

Elimination of Wastes

Svedavaha Srotas is the channel system that is the vehicle for the movement of sweat and the sebaceous fluids. Its origin is adipose tissue, skin, and hair follicles. *Mutravaha Srotas* is the channel system that transports urine. Its origin is the kidneys and urinary bladder. *Purishavaha Srotas* or *Varcovaha Srotas* is the channel system that carries the feces. Its origin is the colon and the rectum.

Mental Functioning

Manovaha Srotas is the channel system that is correlated to mentation, thinking as well as mood and emotions. Its material origin is considered to be in nerve tissue. The "mental" aspect of this system is termed *Manas* (mind) and is connected to the *Majjavaha Srotas* and the *Shukravaha Srotas* in a special way. Mental experience, per se, is considered to be more closely tied in with the *Manomaya Kosha* or mental sheath that exists on the subtle energetic level of the individual's total makeup.

Female Functioning

Artavavaha Srotas or *Rajavaha Srotas* is the system of channels that are involved in menstruation and, in part, some reproductive functions and sexual secretory products. Its origin is the uterus. *Stanyavaha Srotas* is the channel system relating to lactation and to carrying breast milk. Its origin is the uterus.

AGNI: THE DIGESTIVE, METABOLIC FIRE

The concept of *Agni* is central in Ayurveda. References to it are found in the ancient Vedic texts, especially *Rig-Veda* and *Athara-Veda*. In the latter, *Agni* is described as a destroyer of demons and diseases; in addition, it is seen as the body's capacity to replenish the muscle tissue that has been destroyed by external factors. *Agni* is viewed as the power of transformation and as the mediator between the macrocosm (*Brahmanda*) and man (*Pinda*). *Agni* is characterized by various qualities: upward mobility, fragrance, heat, dryness, and lightness. The feature of upward mobility in *Agni* is considered its prime attribute.

Agni, ontologically positioned on the subtle, ethereal, or energetic plane, is situated in the whole body but especially in the functional aspects of the *Pitta dosha. Agni* works through the medium of *Pitta.* Whereas *Agni* as a subtle force controls all metabolic processes in the body, it is regarded as the digestive fire itself, and as such is traditionally understood as a dry and upwardly flowing energy. The *Pitta* in the body is regarded as a coarser or more material substance that acts chiefly as the container of *Agni,* and as such is more liquid and able to flow in all directions. This digestive *Pitta* is usually understood as the functioning of the subdosha, *Pachaka Pitta,* the *Pitta* of the small intestine. *Ranjaka Pitta* is the *Agni* of metabolism.

The body *Agni* (*deha Agni*) has the following associations:

1. *Ayu*: with life
2. *Varna*: with the complexion
3. *Bala*: with physical strength
4. *Utsaha*: with dynamism
5. *Upchaya*: with physical build
6. *Prabha*: with the body's luster
7. *Ojas*: with the body's vitality
8. *Swastha*: with health
9. *Prana*: with the Pranic energy of the breath

Digestion

Agni is most intimately identified with the entire process of digestion. *Agni* is present and active in the body from the cellular level to the more complex levels of tissues and organs. This concept of *Agni* and digestion extends to include transformations and processing that also occur in the psychological domains of thinking and feeling. *Agni,* therefore, is the active principle of transformation that operates on all five sheaths that make up each individual in his entirety: (1) *Annamaya kosha*, the physical sheath; (2) *Pranamaya kosha*, the breath sheath; (3) *Manomaya kosha*, the mental-emotional sheath; (4) *Vijnanomaya kosha*, the wisdom-intelligence sheath; and (5) *Anandamaya kosha*, the bliss sheath. The optimal functioning of *Agni* is directly related to the optimal quality of one's life on all levels and includes the physical, psychological, subtle, and consciousness. The description and functioning of the digestive *Agni* is threefold: (1) *Jatharagni*, the primary digestive metabolic fire that occurs in the gastrointestinal tract; (2) *Bhutagni*, which includes the digestive transformations that are related to the processing of the five Elements in the liver; and (3) *Dhatuagni*, which includes the digestive and metabolic processes within the *dhatus* or tissues.

The processing of nutrition is one of *Agni's* central functional roles. This has two important components: (1) handling the six primary tastes (*rasa*) that Ayurveda identifies within any ingested substance, and (2) facilitating the assimilation of each of the five primary Elements within a food or herb. An extensive discussion of *rasa* as "taste" in the Ayurvedic view will be found in a separate chapter.

Jatharagni and Primary Digestion

Jatharagni is the primary digestive fire located in the lower part of the stomach and in the small intestine. There is only one *Jatharagni* and it is closely allied to *Pachaka Pitta*. Food (*ahara*) that enters the mouth becomes processed into one uniform suspension known as *ahara rasa*. This primary digestive process, the initial or preparatory processing of food, is composed of two parts: (1) *Avasthapaka*, also termed *Prapaka*; and (2) *Vipaka*, the postdigestive effect.

Avasthapaka

Avasthapaka has three phases: (1) *Kapha* or the sweet phase; (2) *Pitta* or the sour phase; and (3) *Vata* or the pungent phase.

The *Kapha* or sweet phase begins in the mouth under the influence of the *Bodhaka Kapha*. It is dominated by the sweet taste. As food descends into the esophagus and reaches the stomach, the alkaline and heavier secretions of the *Kledaka Kapha* continue the frothification and "humidifying" digestive action. In the stomach, the Earth and the Water Elements are digested and absorbed.

The *Pitta* or sour phase begins after about 90 minutes in the lower part of the stomach and in the small intestine by the action of the *Pachaka Pitta*. The sour taste predominates. The *Pittas* of the liver and pancreas heavily contribute to this digestive phase. In this main digestive stage, the Fire Element is digested and absorbed.

The *Vata* or pungent phase begins about 4 hours after the initial ingestion of food and takes place in the large intestine. This is dominated by a pungent taste caused by the action of the *Apana* subdosha of *Vata*. The Air and Ether Elements are considered to be digested and absorbed here. Waste materials are also processed in this phase. The undigested portion of the Earth Element is discarded as feces. In addition to the usable portion of water and minerals that are absorbed, indigestible portions are also reabsorbed and traverse the body to collect other wastes (*kleda*) in its journey to the kidneys for ultimate excretion. The purest aspects of the Air Element that contain *Prana* are absorbed into the body; unusable Air is expelled.

Vipaka: The Postdigestive Effect

The conception of *Vipaka*, the postdigestive effect of food, is unique to Ayurveda. *Vipaka* refers to the delayed and whole body, systemic effect exerted by each of the six tastes (sweet, sour, salty, bitter, pungent, astringent) of a food or an herb. *Vipaka* denotes the actual assimilation of nutrients into cells and tissues. It is a kind of microdigestive process that contrasts with and complements the macrodigestive actions that take place in *Avastapaka*. *Vipaka* is the dynamic action, the point of contact, wherein *Agni* sparks the unique assimilative transformation of nutrients into the tissue cells. This is the juncture at which what was previously the "not self" transmutes to become the human *Ahamkara*, a profound identification with and humanization of the outside world to become one with man.

Vipaka has a long-term effect on the *doshas*. Since the effects of *Vipaka* occur and are generalized throughout the entire body, there is no one specific site of action. The end results of *Vipaka,* however, are more circumscribed than those of *Avasthapaka.* Whereas in primary digestion, each of the six primary tastes of food produces a different digestive effect, in *Vipaka* only three resulting taste phases with metabolic effects are produced. This viewpoint, generally held today, was first described by Charaka (c. 700 B.C.) in his ancient medical treatise *Charaka Samhita.* The three taste phases are: (1) the sweet phase; (2) the sour phase; and (3) the pungent phase. A short time thereafter, Sushruta (c. 600 B.C.), in his medical text *Sushruta Samhita,* described the *Vipaka* concept but emphasized only two nutritive end results: (1) *brimhana,* the building up of tissue substance; and (2) *langhana,* the catabolic breakdown of bodily substance.

The sweet *Vipaka* phase results when either the sweet or the salty taste has been ingested. This results in an increase of saliva and the alkaline secretions of the stomach. The primary metabolic effect is one of nutrition and the building up of the body's tissues. Nutritive aspects of *Kapha* are primarily increased. Ayurvedic tonic foods and herbs most often have a sweet *Vipaka.* In addition, the elimination of waste products is enhanced.

The sour *Vipaka* phase results when the sour taste has been ingested. This increases acid and bile secretions in the stomach. Although not as highly nutritious as in the sweet phase, the sour phase produces some nutrition for all the body's tissues, especially the plasma, with the exception of the reproductive tissue. Nutritive *Kapha* is chiefly produced. The elimination of waste products is also enhanced.

The pungent *Vipaka* phase results when the bitter, astringent, and pungent tastes are ingested. This phase is not considered to be useful for either nutrition or for elimination. *Vata* may be increased, at times, and *Kapha* may be reduced. The therapeutic actions of medicinal herbs, however, can be enhanced. This knowledge of foods and herbs that have a pungent *Vipaka* becomes useful in recommending proper dietary regimes and in selecting therapeutically efficacious herbal remedies.

Bhutagni

Bhutagni refers to the five Elemental digestive fires that reside in the liver. They are closely related to the activity of *Ranjaka Pitta*. After the *ahara rasa* is produced from the *Avasthapaka* process of primary digestion, it travels to the liver for a critical transformation. The *ahara rasa* is considered a nonhomologous or nonhuman *Ahamkara* collection of "food" having the five primary Elements in an initially raw, unassimilable state. It is regarded as unprocessed (*asamskara*). The primary function of the *Bhutagnis* is to transmute the unhomologous primary pentads into the homologous or "humanized" Elements that may become part of the human *rasa* or plasma. The *Bhutagnis*, therefore, function like a humanizing *Ahamkara* stamp to transform materials, such as foods and herbs, which have their own nonhuman identity, into the *rasa* that is qualitatively human and, thus, capable of being optimally utilized.

This qualitative transformation is essential for the digestive process, especially *vipaka*, to continue in the balanced and healthy production of the tissues. The *Bhutagnis* also play another critical role in providing the five sensory organs with their respective primary Element in order to enhance their structural integrity and to promote their healthy functioning. If *Ahamkara* fails to properly stamp the Elements within the dietary inputs with its individualized and human identity, then these raw inputs remain raw and are not absorbed as nutrients. They become toxic and are referred to as *Ama*. This has critical significance for health and disease. The more *Ama* produced, the more difficult it is for the individual's innate *Ahamkara* and intuitive sense to discriminate what further materials in the environment would be best to take in. The faulty functioning of *Manas* thus prevails and wrong choices are made. This further increases *Ama* and leads to a vicious cycle until some corrective action is taken to dispel the accumulated toxins and restore *Ahamkara* to a more balanced state enabling the individual to make healthier choices for his particular constitutional needs.

Dhatuagni: Secondary Digestion or Tissue Metabolism

Dhatuagni is tissue metabolism and digestion. *Dhatuagni* is also referred to as the *tissue fire, tissue metabolism* of the *srotas*, and as *secondary digestion*. Tissue metabolism occurs within the *dhara kala* (containing, nutritive, and metabolic membrane), specific for each particular tissue *srotas* or tissue channel system. The primary site for this is in the liver.

There are seven *Dhatuagnis* that produce their respective tissue elements (*dhatus*) and their respective waste products (*dhatus malas* and *kleda*). They are: (1) *rasadhatuagni;* (2)*raktadhatu-agni;* (3) *mamsadhatuagni;* (4) *medadhatuagni;* (5) *asthidhatuagni;* (6) *majjadhatuagni;* and (7) *shukradhatuagni.*

THE FIVE ELEMENTS AND THE RESPECTIVE TISSUES THEY NOURISH

The five Elements are conceptually regarded both as material building blocks and as representing physiological functions. This dual aspect is reflected in their contribution to the makeup of the bodily tissues, and overall bodily structure and functioning.

1. The Earth Element is the primary material that is the basis for the body's nutrition and bulk. The protein of the body in the form of muscle is fed by the Earth Element.
2. The Water Element contributes to plasma, blood, reproductive fluids, and fat tissue.
3. The Fire Element contributes to the digestive enzymes, hydrochloric acid, and hemoglobin.
4. The Air Element contributes to the buildup of bone and nerves.
5. The Ether Element contributes to the nutrition of the five senses and to the mind.

AMA: METABOLIC TOXIN

A fundamental concept in Ayurveda is that of *Ama,* which generally refers to metabolic toxins or impurities. The word *Ama* is derived from the Sanskrit root *am* which means to harm and to weaken. Along with the optimal production of the end products of digestion that contribute to the overall health and nutrition of the body, there is usually a simultaneous and ongoing buildup of *Ama*. *Ama* results from less than optimal digestion, and this is the usual rather than the exceptional case even in essentially healthy individuals. Improper eating habits, poor food choices, seasonal and lifestyle factors all contribute to impairments of the digestive process and the production of *Ama*, which constitutes an array of metabolic impurities. *Ama* is considered a metabolic toxin since it represents the incomplete or undigested portion of food that becomes nonassimilable yet materially present in the gastrointestinal tract. Vitiated *doshas*, particularly *Vata*, propel (*prakupita*) *Ama* into the circulation and into the tissues. *Ama* acts as a toxic, virtually "foreign" mass within the tissues. It has a propensity to seek out and then deposit itself in weakened and devitalized body tissues. This becomes the ground for future disease processes. The central factor that determines whether *Ama* will be produced is the healthy or impaired state of *Agni*, the digestive fire.

FOUR CONDITIONS OF THE BODY'S *AGNI*

An individual's *Agni* is a function of his or her individual constitution or body type (*prakruti*). *Agni* may also be disturbed intermittently as a result of daily and seasonal intervening factors as was previously mentioned, i.e., diet, lifestyle, weather, etc. Four functional conditions of the *Agni* are recognized: (1) *Sama Agni*, balanced *Agni*; (2) *Tikshna Agni*, high *Agni*; (3) *Mandagni*, low Agni; and (4) *Vishama Agni*, variable *Agni*.

The Ayurvedic system strives to achieve and maintain *Sama Agni*. The condition of impaired *Agni*, however, is the more usual finding. *Mandagni* is commonly found in individuals with *Kapha* predominance, constitutional types characterized by a large frame, tendency toward overweight, consistent appetite, good endurance, and an overall tendency toward stability and possible lethargy. *Tikshna Agni* is found in *Pitta* predominant persons. These individuals have medium frames, average body weight, strong appetites, compelling drive, and competitive and directive personality styles. *Vishama Agni* is seen in those who tend toward the *Vata* constitution characterized by irregularity and unevenness in both physical and psychological areas but adept at spontaneity and creativity.

Lastly, it would not be an overstatement to say that *Agni,* in truth, is more than just the digestive fire. *Agni* is the very *flame of life.* It is the physiologic fire that keeps the body warm and in a constant state of active metabolic transformation. *Agni* not only controls the body's temperature; it is the body's temperature. Akin to the concept of *virya,* the energetic potency of substances, *Agni* maintains the optimal, functional heating of the entire body. This includes proper temperature regulation in order to limit the inordinate proliferation of *krimi,* the ancient Sanskrit term referring to bacteria, viruses, fungi, parasites, and other infectious organisms. In its more concrete forms, *Agni* energizes and exerts its actions through the five subdoshas of *Pitta.* The ingestion of food ignites *Agni,* and this, in turn, activates the workings of *Pitta,* especially in the processes of digestion, metabolism, and transformation.

CHAPTER 5

PRAKRUTI AND *VIKRUTI*

PRAKRUTI: CONSTITUTIONAL TYPE

The Ayurvedic conceptualization of individual, constitutional body types or *prakruti* is a cornerstone of basic theory and practical application (Svoboda, 1989). The term *prakruti* is identical with the term *Prakriti;* both mean first creation. To differentiate their pragmatic use in the Ayurvedic system, they are here spelled differently. *Prakriti* is the metaphysical concept that refers to the primordial, first, and continual stirrings within the Absolute, the *Purusha,* that initiate the beginnings of all the rest of the created world. The word *prakruti* specifically refers to the unique psychophysiological constitution of a specific individual person. The individual *prakruti* expresses itself as a person's body type, that is, as the expression of his or her own individual genetic code. An individual's *prakruti* determines how the varieties of matter that structure the body and the energies that regulate its functioning are handled. The *prakruti* reflects an inborn metabolic pattern, the strength, weakness, and trends that the genetic equipment produces. *Prakruti* is intimately allied with *Agni,* the core template determining an individual's transformative and metabolic code.

In a psychological sense, understanding of the self, so to speak, is equated with an understanding of one's *prakruti.* To maintain overall mental and physical health, one must know one's *prakruti.* Knowing which *doshas* predominate in the constitution permits one to select an array of proper life choices (*pathya*) that include compatible foods, lifestyle activities, exercise, and career that will not aggravate or unduly increase naturally dominant body *doshas*. The usual guidelines suggest incorporating things with opposite doshic qualities, therefore maintaining balance of the *doshas* and of the *prakruti*.

Ayurveda firmly adheres to the proposition that each person, though sharing common human characteristics, is essentially a unique creation, a "first creation." The use of the concept *prakruti*, therefore, is a fractal dimension of the concept of *Prakriti*; it connotes the property of complex self-similarity and implies the understanding that all of reality operates ontologically as series of dynamic, cyclic repetitions. The individual *prakruti* is as significant as the cosmic *Prakriti*; both are first creations yet on different scales in time and space. The concept of normality, in this view, sets the individual as his own standard. An individual is considered normal to the extent that his *prakruti* is functioning in a balanced and optimal manner according to its own unique, inherent configuration.

Individual *prakruti* is established at conception and during the gestation process. Four main factors contribute to it: (1) *shukra beej*, the paternal genes; (2) *artav beej*, the maternal genes; (3) *ksheta* and *garbhashaya*, the state of the mother's womb and her nutrition (*ambu*); and (4) *ritu* or *rutu*, the season of the year. Some Ayurvedic schools of thought differentiate the unalterable *prakruti* established at birth (*janma prakruti*) from the developed and later stabilized *prakruti* (*deha prakruti*) found in adulthood.

The genetic contributions of the parents contain varying amounts and combinations of the influence of the three *doshas*, *Vata*, *Pitta*, *Kapha* (VPK), as well as definite proportions of both the primary Elements (Ether, Air, Fire, Water, Earth) and the *Maha gunas* (*Sattva*, *Rajas*, *Tamas*). When the *prakruti* of an individual is set, it then has a relatively stable arrangement of the VPK principles. This established composition of the doshic principles is the individual's *prakruti*, which determines that individual's particular physiologic mechanisms for energy regulation. For example, some may have a predominance of the *Vata* (propulsion) principle and only very small amounts of the *Pitta* (transformation) and *Kapha* (consolidation) doshic principles. This *prakruti*, therefore, would be called a *Vata prakruti*. If there were a predominance of *Pitta* and *Kapha* with a very small amount of *Vata*, then that *prakruti* would be called a *Pitta/Kapha prakruti*. Although each person has some of all three *doshas* in the *prakruti*, usually one or two *doshas* predominate. The resultant set *prakruti* combination, while relatively constant, will undergo the natural cyclic changes of relative increase and relative decrease of component *doshas* depending on diet, lifestyle, stress, season, and intercurrent illness. The actual possible combinations are numerous. It would not be an exaggeration to state that, in fact, there are as many individual *prakrutis* as there are individuals. In general, however, seven basic types of *prakruti* are commonly found. They are: (1) *Vata*; (2) *Pitta*; (3) *Kapha*; (4) *Vata/Pitta*; (5) *Pitta/Kapha*; (6) *Vata/Kapha*; and (7) *Vata/Pitta/Kapha*.

The concept of *prakruti* has both morphological and functional implications. Since *prakruti* denotes one's body type and constitution, the physical appearance, structure, and innate metabolic tendencies that are produced contribute in characteristic ways to the instinctive responses elicited in the individual by all varieties of external and internal stimuli. The *prakruti* determines, in part, an individual's attraction to sensory inputs, food, ideas, etc. In addition, *prakruti* shapes how these are taken in and processed both physically and psychologically. The *prakruti* has been called one's "first nature." This connotes the given and reflexive response of the individual to the environment. It may have negative consequences over the course of time since growth, maturation, and development change with varying environmental situations. An Ayurvedic understanding of *prakruti*, which includes a correct recognition of real needs and how to address them, produces what has been called one's "second nature." This "second nature" may be thought of as one's intelligently developed capacity to manage the more undisciplined and reflexive inclinations of one's "first nature."

In Ayurveda, the individual is considered to have an innate faculty for correct discrimination, the *Buddhi* aspect of one's makeup. The body (*sthula sharira*) tends toward responding in this innately correct manner. The errors, mistakes, and impairments in judgment, however, that usually prevail, are a function of *Manas* or mind. Mind, in this sense, refers to the more undisciplined and indiscriminately pleasure-seeking human proclivity. The system of Ayurveda assists in educating one to be cognizant of all these issues and influences. Taming the mind and developing the powers of intelligent discrimination follow from this. One's *prakruti* or constitutional predilection, therefore, does not absolutely predetermine preferences and subsequent doshic balances or imbalances. *Prakruti* sets a psychophysiologic tone that can be modulated by the experiential interactions of itself and the environment. Although one's *prakruti* has innate characteristic proclivities, the ability to selectively choose different options such as foods or lifestyle habits permits one to experience considerable flexibility in daily living.

Constitutional Characteristics

Prakruti is made up of varying mixes of *Vata, Pitta,* and *Kapha* and one's unique *prakruti* reflects the varying qualities inherent in that constitutional doshic type. *Prakruti* may be thought of as having three basic domains of expression: (1) physical; (2) cognitive; and (3) psychological. Since all *prakruti* types contain some degree of all three *doshas*, and since the doshic predominance may not contain every one of its characteristic properties, there is a gradation of overall *prakruti* expression. With this in mind, a general outline of *prakruti* conformations will be examined.

Vata Predominant *Prakruti*

Vata prakruti has the basic attributes of *Vata dosha*: cold, dry, light, subtle, mobile and erratic, sharp and quick, hard, rough, and clear. The physical characteristic associated with those having *Vata* predominance are tendencies toward thin bodies, small frames, protuberant and cracking joints, crooked or uneven teeth, small eyes, cold limbs, and dry skin. The variable and irregular metabolism characteristic of *Vata* types contributes to this. Sleep may be light and of brief duration. Physical activity is irregular and may run in spurts of excess versus little activity. There may be restlessness and low stamina. The quality of the voice may be breathy and its strength weak. *Vata* types are usually very talkative. There is difficulty falling and staying asleep.

Appetite and digestion are irregular, as well, and there is a tendency toward constipation. There is a preference for warmer climates and an aversion toward cold. Body odor and sweating are minimal. Women may have irregular menstrual cycles. Sex drive and libido are said to be characterized by much imagination, intermittent excesses, and lower than average fertility. In contrast to the other doshic types, there is a significantly greater susceptibility to disease, and lifespan is believed to be relatively shorter. Disease manifestations tend to include pain, arthritis, and proneness to mental disorders.

The cognitive characteristics of *Vata* include exceptional alertness, and quick, active mental functioning. New ideas are quickly grasped, but just as quickly forgotten.

The psychological characteristics of the *Vata* constitution include creativity, freshness, and enthusiasm. *Vata* types are sensitive, high strung, changeable, fidgety, impulsive, and restless. They may have tendencies toward anxiety and fear. Many new activities are launched, but since concentration is usually mobile and difficult to sustain, they often fail to complete an endeavor. Lastly, there is a tendency toward ambivalence and indecisiveness.

Pitta Predominant *Prakruti*

Pitta prakruti has attributes characteristic of *Pitta dosha*: hot, slightly oily, light, subtle, mobile and steady, sharp and penetrating, soft, smooth, clear, and flowing. The physical characteristics of *Pitta prakruti* include moderate body build, fair or reddish and warm complexion, thin and sparse hair, and a tendency toward having skin moles and freckles. Appetite is usually strong and digestion is good. There may be problems with gastric hyperacidity. Bowel movements are regular but may be loose; at times, *Pitta*'s heat may produce constipation. Sleep is sound and of medium duration. There is a tendency toward sweating and more pronounced body odor. There is an aversion to warm and humid weather and a preference for the cold. Sexual desire is moderate and its gratification can be well modulated; fertility is average. Lifespan is believed to be moderate.

Disease proneness includes manifestations of inflammatory conditions, fevers, hyperacidity, hypertension, and liver and blood problems.

The cognitive characteristics of *Pitta* include a sharp, penetrating intellectual faculty with little ambivalence. *Pitta* types tend to be well organized, methodical, and managerial in style.

The psychological characteristics of *Pitta* types include bold, focused, courageous, and intense outlooks with strong leadership qualities. There is a tendency toward competitiveness and critical judgment. Being demanding, having an irritable temper, and a quality of wanting to be dominant prevail.

Kapha Predominant *Prakruti*

Kapha prakruti has properties of the *Kapha dosha*: cold, damp, heavy, coarse, compact, dull, soft, smooth, sticky, and dense. Physical characteristics include solid, heavy body build, good musculature, a tendency toward overweight and subcutaneous fat, soft and oily skin, thick dark wavy hair, large soft eyes, and big uniform pearl white teeth. Appetite is hearty, digestion is slow, and elimination is regular. Although there is a pronounced tendency toward lethargy and laziness, physical stamina is excellent, as is general health. There is a tendency to sleep a great deal; sleep is heavy and deep. There is an aversion for cool, damp climates. *Kapha prakruti* experiences steady sexual desire that can be felt as strong and capable of sustained arousal; fertility is usually excellent. Lifespan is believed to be very long. Disease proneness includes manifestations of respiratory disorders, edema, hypercholesterolemias, obesity, and tumors.

Cognitive characteristics reflect a slowness to learn but very good long-term memory. Intellectual pursuits are not especially sought since learning requires effort and repetition, which is not characteristic of the *Kapha* style.

The psychological characteristics of *Kapha prakruti* include a calm, tranquil, and steady mode. There is a great deal of patience, perseverance, and compassion. They tend to be generous, affectionate, loving, forgiving, conservative, and loyal. Speech is clear and unhurried; voice is deep and melodious. In excess, *Kapha* types tend toward possessiveness, attachment, greed, depression, and lethargy.

Vata/Pitta Prakruti

Vata/Pitta prakruti shares characteristics of both of its *doshas*. Build may be slightly more muscular than that of the sinewy *Vata* person. They may be gregarious, friendly, and talkative. Digestion is good with more of a quality of regularity. The possible *Vata* motivated tendency toward addiction may express itself as self-medicating with prescribed or illicit drugs; this may be enhanced by the *Pitta* tendency toward wishing to intensify experiences. There is an energetic and more focused quality to their daily activities.

Pitta/Kapha Prakruti

This *prakruti* favorably combines the penetrating sharpness of the *Pitta* with the stability and evenness of the *Kapha dosha*. Body build is more muscular and solid. Energy level is high and sustainable. There may be a tendency, however, to overconfidence.

Vata/Kapha Prakruti

The *Vata/Kapha* may be quick and efficient as well as steady and determined in a more regular fashion. There may be some impairment of digestion because of a predominance of the cold attribute common to both *Vata* and *Kapha* as well as a marked intolerance of cold climates.

Vata/Pitta/Kapha Prakruti

This triple *dosha* type is termed the *sama prakruti*. When in balance, this *prakruti* has the optimal characteristics of all three *doshas*. This constitutional type, however, is not common.

Finer Distinctions of *Prakruti*

The basic conceptualization of *prakruti*, however apparently simple, is not, in fact, simplistic. There are finer degrees of differentiation that take into account aspects of the individual across the metaphysical–physical spectrum.

Physical *Prakruti* and the Five Elements

Prakruti as described so far has taken into consideration the gross or physical body since constitutional type usually refers to the doshic composition that reflects specific physiologic tendencies. The structural and morphological constitution of the physical body is understood in more detailed fashion from the perspective of the *Pancha Mahabhutanis*, the five great gross Elements (Ether, Air, Fire, Water, and Earth). The Ayurvedic conceptualization of the Elements, it is to be remembered, goes beyond a denotation of their being merely groupings of material atoms. It includes their additional transcendent operations consisting of a host of implicit innate trends that impart characteristic and enduring form, content, and functional traits to the substances that they compose. Each individual has a predominance of one or more of the primary pentads, the five great Elements. Each one of the pentadic Elements is associated with distinctive characteristics that are more apparent on the physical, material level although these Elements also impart psychological characteristics as well. It is to be remembered that the individual *doshas*, themselves, are combinations of specific primary Elements. *Vata* is composed of a predominance of Ether and Air; *Pitta* has a predominance of Fire and Water; and *Kapha* has a predominace of Water and the Earth Element.

Akasha, or the Ether Element, is associated with large, spacious, and grand characteristics. Very large physical features such as excessively large ears or bone structure, for instance, suggest a predominance of Ether in the body. Large, external body openings such as the ears, the eyes, and the nostrils are characteristic of the Ether Element. Those who have a predominance of Ether have internal organs that are well differentiated; their internal body spaces, the thoracic and abdominal cavities, for example, may be large. The intercellular spaces may occupy more area. This greater spatial configuration contributes to an increased potential for movement and change. Hearing and sound sensitivities are associated with Ether and so are more prominent as is the strength of the speech faculty. Weak areas in the makeup of the body include the tendency for dilatation potentially manifesting in cardiac (congestive heart failure) and in lung problems (emphysema). Tinnitus of the ears may also be present. Psychological qualities that are expansive, highly intuitive, and reflect high values and moral standards are also characteristic, especially since the sattvic *guna* is predominant. The sattvic *guna,* or *Sattva,* is the innate tendency in *Prakriti,* creation in all its manifestations, toward purity, balance, coherence, intelligence, and spirituality.

Vayu, or the Air Element, is associated with a great deal of mobility, dynamism, and amorphousness. Physical appearance manifests complexions that are light, pink, dry, and rough. The skin may be thin and show prominent blood vessels, tendons, and joints. There is a characteristic popping sound to the joints commonly referred to as "cracking of the joints." Those with a predominance of the Air Element may be particularly motorically active and may become easily exhausted. Their sleep is light. In addition to being easily distractible, potential weaknesses include susceptibility to the cold, various neuromuscular disorders, neuralgia, arthritis, and a tendency to constipation. *Prana* and *Vayu* are intimately related and produce a well-developed sense of touch and a talent for healing. The rajasic *guna* is active in this Element. *Rajas* is the *Maha guna* within *Prakriti* that is associated with turbulence, stimulation, and activity.

Tejas or *Agni,* the Fire Element, is associated with transformation, change, conversion, and visual perception. Intensity and penetration are associated with a predominance of this Element. Those with a *Tejas* predominance appear bright, light, and may have complexions with a pinkish hue. They do not tolerate heat well, and have light but sound sleep. They are highly intelligent, organized, managerial, competitive, somewhat impatient, and strive for success and achievement. When ill, they suffer from inflammatory conditions, hyperacidity, ulcers, hypertension, and are prone to hematological disorders. Their sense of sight is particularly acute. *Sattva* and *Rajas* are the *Maha gunas* that predominate.

Ap or *Jala*, the Water Element, is characterized by features that are liquid, flowing, and capable of taking on multiple forms without losing its identity. Those with a Water Element predominance appear to have light and fair complexions with bodies that are soft, smooth, somewhat "chubby," and cool to the touch. Their hair is soft and wavy; they appear well nourished and "moist." They are particularly affectionate and loving, and their sexual drive is strong. The sensory faculty of taste may be acutely developed. When out of balance, they are prone to congestive disorders such as colds, sinus difficulties, and asthma. They may develop edema and diabetic conditions. *Rajas* and *Tamas* are dominant. *Tamas* is the *Maha guna* associated with inertia, cohesion, density, and materiality.

Prithvi, the Earth Element, is a solid, dense, rigid, and relatively inert substance. This manifests in a physical appearance that is "earthy" with large, heavy muscular and bone development. The complexion may tend to be dark. Although their general demeanor is slow and somewhat lethargic, they tend to be calm and stable. They have a need for more than an average amount of sleep. Those with a dominant Earth Element tend to be forgiving and capable of deep and lasting attachments. With such a strong complement of the most material Element, there is a susceptibility to tumors of bone and muscle. The olfactory sense may be particularly well developed. These persons are more tamasic in nature. *Tamas* is dominant.

Psychological *Prakruti* and the *Maha gunas*

The predominance of the quality of one or more of the three *Maha gunas* (*Sattva, Rajas, Tamas*) at the time of birth contributes to the psychological constitution of the individual. The *Maha gunas* can never exist singly in nature; they are always present in differing admixtures and this gives infinite variety to the substances they imbue. Nuances of temperament and overall character style are virtually unlimited and defy adequate classification. A general description of the key attributes of various subdivisions of the major three doshic constitutions will be given, however, in order to suggest an approximate understanding of the Ayurvedic notion of some psychological *prakruti* types. Sattvic (pure) qualities are primary and foster movement toward increased consciousness. Rajasic (turbulence) and tamasic (dulling) qualities, significant, necessary, and modulating as they are, tend to be less consciousness enhancing.

Vata Psychological *Prakruti*

The sattvic complement provides a positive energy with features that include harmony, equilibrium, adaptability, strong healing qualities, quick comprehension, and a general sense of cheerfulness, happiness, and freshness. This is the mental domain closest to pure consciousness. The rajasic component, although providing the driving force of enthusiasm, fresh creation, and novelty, may create, at times of imbalance, a disturbing overall dynamic that includes features of anxiety, insecurity, agitation, volatility, explosiveness, impulsivity, inattention, indecisiveness, mania, loquaciousness, oppositional behavior, irresponsibility, and insomnia. The tamasic *Maha guna,* in states of imbalance, may tend to produce fear, depression, dishonesty, boredom, and proneness to drug addiction, sexual perversion, and other mental disturbances.

Pitta Psychological *Prakruti*

The sattvic complement creates discriminating intelligence (*prajna*), clarity of consciousness, sound judgment, harmony, courage, organizational proficiency, self-discipline, will power, and leadership. The rajasic *Maha guna* can introduce turbulence, competitiveness, ambitious and dominating tendencies, manipulation, irritability, defiance, inordinate anger, envy, pride, narcissism, and lustful desire. Likewise, in a state of imbalance, the tamasic component may elicit hate, violence, destructiveness, and a proneness to criminal activities.

Kapha Psychological *Prakruti*

The sattvic *guna* creates a quality of harmony, calm, serenity, peace of mind, compassion (*karuna*), devotion, nurturance, loving, devotion, the ability to forgive, stability, and strength. The rajasic component may enhance the qualities of inordinate attachment, materialism, greed, greedy lustfulness, and jealousy. The tamasic component can produce inordinate coarseness, lethargy, sloth, dull comprehension, apathy, boredom, procrastination, and severe depression.

Ancient Ayurvedic Classification of Psychological *Prakruti*

Ancient Ayurvedic texts describe seven types of sattvic *prakruti,* six rajasic types, and three tamasic types. This sort of typing is not commonly done in initial assessments nowadays. A very brief description, which is of historical interest, however, is as follows.

1. Sattvic *prakruti* types: Brahma *prakruti* demonstrates characteristics of purity, sincerity, respect, and intelligence. *Mahendra prakruti* shows courage, obedience, and devotion. *Varuna prakruti* has pleasing conversation, is tolerant, and prefers cold. *Kaubera prakruti* is skilled at accumulating wealth, and implementing ideas. *Gandharva prakruti* appreciates beauty, dance, and fine fragrances. *Yama prakruti* is fearless, pure, observant of propriety, and shows mental equanimity. *Asra prakruti* demonstrates balanced intellectual and spiritual development; it reflects responsible, faithful, and disciplined behavior.
2. Rajasic *prakruti* types: *Asura prakruti* is solitary, somewhat hedonistic, and intimidating. *Sarpa prakruti* is intelligent but may be deceitful and deceptive. *Sakuna prakruti* shows volatility, anger, and overindulgence in eating and sexual behavior. *Raksasa prakruti* shows anger, envy, irreligiosity, and arrogance. *Paisaca prakruti* is bold, daring, amorous, and lacking in shame. *Praita prakruti* is selfish, greedy, lazy, and irritable.
3. Tamasic *prakruti* types: *Pasava prakruti* is dull, sluggish, and unable to follow directions. *Matysa prakruti* is unwise, cowardly, interpersonally aggressive, and said to be fond of water. *Vanaspatya prakruti* shows vegetative traits such as being sessile, and lacking in attention to the prescribed Vedic goals of *dharma* (responsibility and virtue), *artha* (working for food,

clothing, and shelter), *kama* (healthy enjoyment), and *moksha* (the freedom of self-actualization).

Overall Assessment of *Prakruti*

The evaluation of an individual's *prakruti* constitutes the first step in the Ayurvedic assessment process. *Prakruti* is generally regarded as an estimation of the doshic constitution that regulates metabolic functioning. A more comprehensive analysis yields a spectrum of highly individualized constitutional types that includes anatomical, physiological, and psychological subgroupings. The constitution of the physical body has a predominance of one or more of the primary Elements. This imparts the special qualities characteristic of that Elemental predominance. The constitution reflecting the physiological functioning is determined by *dosha* predominance. This, too, has at its base an underlying dominance of the features of the Elements unique to those respective predominant *doshas*. Through pulse diagnosis, to be discussed later, one may ascertain a subdosha predominance, as well, that would give more specificity to the overall *prakruti* assessment. Lastly, there is a significant psychological dimension to the *prakruti*. The dominance and quality of the *Maha gunas* determine these psychological trends.

Ayurveda recognizes the individuality of each person. A comprehensive analysis of *prakruti* reveals the detailed specificity of the constitution. One finds variations in body type and psychological type, i.e., *Kapha dosha prakruti* with *Manas* having a rajasic and tamasic quality. A person like this, for example, would have a sturdy, well-nourished body, and a mind that was driven at times and lethargic at others. The *prakruti* conception, therefore, should be understood as indicating an operational form that acts as a template or blueprint to process data that come in from the changing environments and subjective states that each individual experiences. This makes for a virtually infinite number of constitutional types and possible responses, and eliminates the idea of a set and rigidly predetermined system.

Sattvic Enhancement

A basic principle in Ayurveda is to foster the development of sattvic (pure) qualities and to regulate the balance of rajasic (turbulent) and tamasic (dulling) tendencies. Sattvic attributes include enhanced, refined consciousness, intelligence, compassion, purity, balance, integration, mental and emotional equanimity, trustfulness, and the inclination toward a healthy lifestyle. To the extent that a simple word might approximate, yet possibly oversimplify, the profound meaning of *Sattva*, the term *goodness* is suggested. Rajasic trends, especially when negative, include the inordinate experience of desire, lust, concupiscence, anger, and cynicism. Tamasic qualities, when devoid of sattvic modulation, tend toward inertia, concreteness, avarice, depression, fear, ignorance, and violence.

VIKRUTI

Prakruti refers to the specific doshic combination that makes up the body type or constitution. When the *prakruti* reflects the healthy, normal functioning of each of its component *doshas* alone and in their combined state, this condition of balance is the condition of health (*swastha*). When the *prakruti* becomes disturbed and the *doshas* qualitatively vitiate, accumulate in excess, decline and become deficient, or interact among themselves negatively, the *prakruti*, now, is referred to as *vikruti*, the imbalanced state of an individual's constitution.

The *vikruti* condition is common, and reflects the rapidly changing state of the *doshas*. These imbalances can result from diet, lifestyle, stress, age, and the seasonal shifts. They may be temporary and last for a few days or weeks, or accumulate over the seasons and last for years. An important aim of Ayurveda is to evaluate the basic *prakruti*, assess the current imbalanced state, the *vikruti*, and restore optimal functioning to each *dosha* and proper balance to the overall functioning of the *doshas* individually and as they interact in combination. The Ayurvedic view of health and disease, health maintenance, disease prophylaxis, and treatment addresses these issues.

CHAPTER 6

HEALTH AND THE DISEASE PROCESS. I

HEALTH AND DISEASE CONCEPTS

The concept of health and well-being (*swastha*) in Ayurveda grounds itself in the idea of fostering the balanced and normal functioning of the *doshas*, that is, restoring the *prakruti* to equilibrium when states of constitutional imbalance (*vikruti*) occur. The optimal functioning of each *dosha* in the body creates a homeostatic condition that is conducive to overall health and well-being. Ayurveda views health as a comprehensive state of balance that includes the optimal quality, quantity, and functioning of the *doshas*, *dhatus* (tissues), *srotas* (channels), *malas* (waste products), *Agni* (digestive fire), and *Ojas* (immune system).

Disease is viewed as a state of imbalance produced by imbalances in the *doshas* and subsequent impairments in the functioning of the *Agni*, the channels, the tissues and organs, waste products, and the immune system. Terms for disease are *roga* and *amaya*. The commonly used term *roga* means that which causes pain and is derived from the Sanskrit root *ruj* meaning *to pain*. The word *duhkha* usually accompanies descriptions of ill health and disease. *Duhkha* is commonly translated as pain with connotations of unpleasantness and pervasive dissatisfaction. The antonym of *duhkha* is *sukha*, which translates as happiness, favorableness, or pleasantness. It is said that Charaka, the renowned Ayurvedic luminary, described disease as the condition in which "ease" is lost. The sense of this is understandable since the root *kha* suggests a space (similar to the notion of Ether or *Akasha*) within the body, and *su* suggests a positive or favorable state, a condition of ease. The term *sukha* implies that bodily spaces such as the channels are in a positive or favorable condition.

The concept of health in Ayurveda also implies the condition of wholeness. This conceptualization has several connotations such as included in the term *samhita* that means integrated compendium, and in the term *advaita* meaning nonduality. Since the medical practice of Ayurveda, as its name implies, derives from the ancient tradition of the *Vedas*, a significant metaphysical dimension of the health concept is fundamental and complements its biological denotation.

The heart of the Ayurvedic concept of health contains the idea that the quality of one's consciousness should reflect wholeness, clarity, coherence, and integration. Consciousness here denotes the most intimate experience of awareness. It goes beyond a merely neurological description of alertness, orientation, and a capacity to concentrate. The definition of disease in the Ayurvedic view would suggest that any condition of impaired consciousness connotes a state of imbalance and some degree of disease, unhappiness, dysphoria, malaise, yearning, and a desire for the satisfaction of unfulfilled needs. This perspective demonstrates the intrinsic spiritual foundation of Ayurvedic thought. Although Ayurveda in theory and in practice places emphasis on the physical dimensions of man, a core spiritual underpinning, consciousness-based, remains its central ballast.

THE THREE UNIVERSAL CAUSES OF ALL DISEASE

Ayurveda describes three common overriding causes that contribute to all disease. They are: (1) *Prajna-aparadha;* (2) *Kala-Parinama;* and (3) *Asatmyendriyartha samyoga.*

Prajna-Aparadha

Prajna-aparadha is a concept that is variously translated as *the mistake of the intellect, volitional transgression,* or *an error in wisdom;* it is the loss of the memory of oneness. This given cognitive blindness is perpetuated, in part, by coercive habit / habituation over time, i.e., repeating the same stereotyped thinking and behaviors in a reflexive, automatic manner without pause, introspection, and contemplative reflection.

Man's manifestation in the material world of flesh and blood constitutes his potential for rediscovering intrinsic unity within diversity by means of efforts toward repair, restoration, and the development of ever-greater expansions of consciousness. This is the meaning of *moksha* (liberation) and *samadhi* (enlightenment). *Prajna-aparadha* is the universal human condition marked by a pervasive neglect or forgetting of the aforementioned interconnectedness of the essential unity of spirit and matter. With the original state of all being considered to be one of pure consciousness, birth into the world makes us oblivious of our origins. Most are distracted by the belief that only the conventionally discernible, material aspects of experience exist and, therefore, must constitute reality in its entirety. The assumption that man is, in fact, an integral composite of matter and spirit in an enormous, almost ineffable, universe of matter and spirit is the underpinning for positing the reality of this cognitive distortion.

In the Ayurvedic view, material realities are not understood as being false or even as "bad." *Prajna-aparadha* maintains an amnesia whose consequences result in forgetting the integrated field of existence, of consciousness at the heart of matter. Ordinary cognition influenced by *Manas* (mind) experiences life as *Viparita-Bhavana,* that is, with the erroneous conviction that the visible world of appearances alone is the only reality. This given condition is explained by the influence of *Manas* on *Buddhi* (the discriminating intellect). Intrinsic to the nature of *Manas* is a dulling of *Buddhi*'s clarity. The epistemological term in Sanskrit for this misinterpretation is called *avidya* and is roughly translated as ignorance. The delusional understanding of reality that results from this becomes formalized in the Sanskrit term *Maya* meaning the world as ordinarily experienced is a grand illusion.

The fundamental significance of *Prajna-aparadha* lies in the fact that the presence of *Manas* tends to produce an incorrect mindset. This is the source of the perversions of desire that repetitively seek pleasure in an almost reflexive fashion. The upshot of this is the ordinary tendency to make wrong and unwholesome choices. In this view, wrong choices are ultimately caused by the puissant influence of *Prajna-aparadha* on the operation of *Manas.* The functioning of *Manas* is virtually synonymous with that of "desire" (*mara, raga*) in almost every sense. What must be clearly understood, if not stressed, is that *Manas,* per se, is not intrinsically bad or evil. *Manas* can be considered our calling card, our ticket of admission, and our key to unlocking our human entry into the manifest world as we ordinarily experience it. In this sense, *Manas* is neutral; it functions as an instrument that provides ample access to a world that can be experienced in perceptual, sensuous, and sensual ways. It provides material that we then are free to process in an unlimited number of ways.

If choices and behaviors that are more wholesome (*satyma*) continually discipline or healthfully shape *Manas,* then the functioning of *Buddhi,* the reality intellect, will be empowered in the overall life of the individual, especially in the physical body (*sthula sharira*). This, in turn, will foster more wholesome, safe, and reality-based choices (*pathya*) that are conducive to health. In this way, listening to the body and addressing its needs yields health; the mind or *Manas,* however, may continue to perpetuate ignorance, hedonistic choice, and thus disease.

Prajna-aparadha is responsible for impairments in the functioning of three important psychological faculties: (1) *dhi;* (2) *dhruti;* and (3) *smruti. Dhi* (wisdom) is the capacity of the *Buddhi* intellect to comprehend the intrinsic laws of nature (*ritam*). *Dhruti* (patience) is the courage to avoid that which is harmful; it implies impulse control and will power. *Smruti* or *smriti* (memory) is the capacity to recall on a continuous basis the activities proper and conducive to health.

Kala-Parinama

Kala-Parinama refers to the transformations produced by the passage of time. This change over time refers to the activity of the *doshas.* When the normal level of a *dosha* is increased, this produces an elevation, potentially unhealthful, in the functioning of that *dosha.* When a *dosha* is decreased, it suggests a less than optimal physiological functioning. Only in the condition of excess, elevated *doshas* and increased doshic functioning, does a tendency toward significant imbalance and disease occur. This encompasses changes that may occur in three ways: (1) over the course of the life cycle; (2) during the course of the day; and (3) during the course of the seasonal shifts of the year.

Doshas and the Life Cycle

According to Ayurveda, the life cycle is divided into three epochs each having a general doshic predominance that acts as an underpinning to the other influences that affect the doshic balance. The period of childhood (*bala*), from birth to adolescence, is the time when *Kapha* (consolidation) predominates. Childhood *Kapha* dominance is associated with the normal processes of growth and the rapid development of the tissues and body structure. *Kapha* imbalances and diseases tend to be respiratory and manifest as colds and as asthma, for example. The period of adolescence (*madhya*) through midlife is considered the epoch of *Pitta* (transformation) predominance. There is a time for refining intellectual and vocational abilities and the display of natural competitiveness as seen in sports, educational, and vocational pursuits. *Pitta*-predominant diseases include inflammatory conditions such as acne, hyperacidity, ulcer, and irritable bowel syndromes, to name just a few. The period of beginning older age (*vriddha*), roughly from about 55 years onward, is the era in which *Vata* (propulsion) predominates. The influence of *Vata* tends to show itself in a broader experiential range of awareness, the "wisdom of older age," and in difficulties such as insomnia, constipation, and arthritis. These age-dependent three different doshic predominances parallel the timing of the maturational, developmental, and hormonal changes that accompany puberty and later menopause and the male climacteric. The three life-cycle divisions and their chronological age correlates, however, are to be understood in a broad sense and only suggest approximations. Individual variations are so common that they take precedence in determining, for instance, the specific age of onset of the older years.

Normal Physiological Diurnal Fluctuations of the *Doshas*

In the course of 24 hours, the three *doshas* regularly cycle and one will predominate over the others. *Kapha* predominates from 6 A.M. to 11 A.M.; *Pitta* predominates from 11 A.M. to 2 P.M.; *Vata* predominates from 2 P.M. to 6 P.M. At this point, the cycle begins again. *Kapha* predominates from 6 P.M. to 11 P.M.; then *Pitta* from 11 P.M. to 2 A.M.; and lastly, *Vata* from 2 A.M. to 6 A.M.

During this normal diurnal cycling, the specific attributes of the *dosha* that predominates hold sway and influence the overall functioning of the body. For example, the early morning *Kapha* predominance is associated with phlegm, water, and other waste product elimination. *Pitta* predominance around noon is associated with increased appetite and normally increased digestive capacity. Ayurveda considers noontime as the best time to have the largest meal of the day.

Normal Seasonal Fluctuations of the *Doshas*

The normal cyclical rise and fall of the bodily *doshas* that is produced by the effect of seasonal changes is a gradual process. The *doshas* are contained in all biological life and this includes the plant world in addition to man and the animals. Varying seasonal conditions act as specific stimuli that elicit doshic reactions in the body. Since man and nature are linked in significantly identificatory ways, both respond accordingly. When qualities and attributes in nature that are *dosha* specific begin to predominate, they elicit a rise in the corresponding *dosha* within man. The seasonal variations in *dosha* predominance have three phases:

1. *Sanchaya,* Accumulation. This phase is one of very gradual accumulation or increase.
2. *Prakopa,* Aggravation or Provocation. During this phase, the particular *dosha* is at an almost maximally increased level.
3. *Prashama,* Alleviation or Pacification. This phase occurs when the previously elevated *dosha* decreases and returns to a more balanced level.

In the United States, there are four seasons: fall, winter, spring, and summer. *Vata* is related to fall and early winter, which is cold and dry. *Kapha* is related to mid- and late winter and to early spring, which is cold and damp. *Pitta* is related to early spring and summer, which is damp and hot. *Vata* begins its gradual accumulation in the summer, and reaches its peak intensity of aggravation in the fall and early winter. In the late winter and spring, when the dry and cold weather becomes more clement, *Vata* is alleviated, the process of a *dosha*'s return to levels that are more physiologically normal for the body. *Pitta* begins its gradual accumulation in the late winter and spring, and reaches its peak intensity in the summer. Summer is the season, therefore, when *Pitta* is provoked and aggravated. When the extreme heat of summer begins to subside as the fall season ensues, increased *Pitta* declines to levels that are more normal, a process referred to as alleviation. *Kapha* gradually accumulates in the fall and early winter, and reaches peak intensity in the late winter and spring. It becomes pacified and alleviated with its normal decline in intensity in the summer.

Asatmyendriyartha Samyoga

The distinctly Ayurvedic concept of *asatmyendriyartha samyoga* can be translated as the unwholesome contact of the sense organs with their sense objects (*vishaya*). The functioning of the sense organs has great significance since it is a central nexus between the individual and the outside world. The five sense organs, the ears, skin, eyes, tongue, and nose, are called the *jnanendriya*, the organs that ingest the objects of sensory perception, the sense objects. When the contact of a sense organ and its object is proper or wholesome (*satyma*), the subtle half of the corresponding primary great Element grasped at that contact point is absorbed. These quanta of energy, the *sukshma Tanmatras*, then go on to feed the more immaterial sheaths (*koshas*) just as actual food and water feeds the physical sheath of the body with the primary Elements. The sense organs, therefore, are the physical vehicles through which the mind (*Manas*) and the discriminating intellect (*Buddhi*), in fact, effect the absorption of the

Tanmatras, the subtle Essences, from experience of the outside world into the energetic dimensions of the individual. This energetic feeding, so to speak, not only replenishes the individual's own store of *Tanmatras*, but the subsequently enhanced *Tanmatras* then go on to produce further vitalization of the body's own primary Elements that, in turn, continue to nourish and replenish the bodily *doshas*, *dhatus* (tissues), etc.

Improper contact of the sense organs with their objects, therefore, is significant since it results in diminished nutritional input on the most subtle, vital levels, with consequential impairment of the interconnected system that affects nutrition on the material tissue level. Improper contact may take three distinct forms: (1) excessive contact; (2) negligible or deficient contact; and (3) unnatural, perverted, or wrong contact.

1. Ear: the sense organ for hearing. Excessive contact consists of listening to harsh sounds, sounds with inordinately high frequencies, or repetitive discordant sounds. Noise pollution, for example, city traffic, motor cycles at high speeds, power tools, and loud machinery represent an array of sounds that may be excessive over a extended period. Prolonged exposure to sound that exceeds 100-decibels (dBA) includes chain saws, snowmobiles, and loud aerobic class environments. Sounds above 110 dBA, considered dangerous by the National Institute on Deafness and Other Communication Disorders, include those produced by firearms, fireworks, jet engines, and also excessively loud concerts and loud music club situations. Negligible contact consists of listening to sounds restricted to only narrow ranges of frequencies, or sensory deprivation of sound input altogether. The concept of negligible contact has been referred to as "insufficient or feeble" contact. Another form of improper contact is defined as exposure to sounds that are irritating and that may be unnatural, such as a sonic boom made by an aircraft or a nuclear explosion, for example. Some Ayurvedic texts refer to this class of improper sensory contact as *perverted*.

2. Skin: the sense organ for tactile sensation. Excessive contact may come from exposure to very rough objects, objects that are of extreme temperatures, or from conditions that are unfavorable over time such as damp or cold climates. Negligible contact results from the absence of adequate massage. Ayurveda

holds that this may constitute a significant impairment, especially for the *Vata dosha*, over the long term. Other wrong contacts involve exposure to irritants such as tobacco smoke, toxic chemicals, and potential carcinogens such as the lead in paint and possibly the ink in some older printing materials, for example.

3. Eye: the sense organ for vision. Excessive contact includes viewing inordinately bright objects, scenes of excessive or violent activity, and exposure to scenes with repetitive, unnatural, and artificial action and themes. Some examples of these include excessive viewing or staring at the sun, explosions, volcanoes, television, the cinema, computer screens, etc. Negligible contact results from remaining in very dark or dim places for prolonged periods. Other forms of wrong contact include viewing objects too closely or from too far a distance. The Ayurvedic literature also describes other examples of improper visual contact by citing the following: viewing frightening animals such as tigers and lions; hideously damaged objects; a solar eclipse; and natural disasters such as destructive floods, earthquakes, etc. The modern world also provides examples of improper or perverted visual contact as, for instance, in exposure to inordinate violence, sexuality, and artificial and natural disasters that are seen in television shows and in the news media. The current psychiatric disorder termed Posttraumatic Stress Disorder can be linked to these.

4. Tongue: sense organ for taste. Excessive contact includes excessive intake of food and drink. Negligible contact refers to eating a disproportionately small quantity and poor quality of food. It also includes the failure to experience through taste the proper complement of the Ayurvedically required nutritional tastes that are necessary for the optimal functioning of the *doshas* in one's *prakruti*. Perverted taste contact refers to eating in a manner (time of day, season, food combinations, etc.) that is contrary to established Ayurvedic dietary guidelines.

5. Nose: sense organ for olfaction. Excessive contact includes contact with overly pungent and irritating smells such as those of chemicals like ammonia and sulphuric acid. Negligible contact includes insufficient contact with pleasing and "nutritionally fortifying" aromas such as those of essential oils that

may be therapeutic and helpful in balancing the *doshas*. Olfactory experience considered wrong includes contact with smells such as those of putrefying material, noxious odors such as poisons, fumes, and pollution from trucks, cars, or aircraft.

AN OVERVIEW OF THE FOUR FUNDAMENTAL MECHANISMS UNDERLYING ALL PATHOGENIC PROCESSES

Disease is a process that occurs over time with multiple contributory factors that have a sequential history. Although all concepts of pathogenesis are complex, the Ayurvedic perspective considers four foundational processes as essential and out of which all disease manifestations occur. They are:

1. *Dosha Utpadaka*, vitiation of the *doshas*
2. *Agnimandya*, impairment of the digestive fire
3. *Ama* formation, metabolic impurities formation
4. *Samprapti*, pathogenesis proper

The Ayurvedic concept of disease emphasizes the idea that the individual becomes ill only when the field of the body, the *doshas* and the *dhatus* (tissues), becomes weakened. This weakened condition is associated with a diminished immunity, lowered resistance to illness, and to lowered *Ojas*, the physical substance that enhances the immune system and pervades the healthy body. Only when specific areas of the tissues are compromised in an appreciable manner can disease actually take hold. Damaged lacunae within the tissues, therefore, become receptive to a variety of causative factors, both internal and external, such as microbes, germs, and infectious processes.

CONCEPT OF *DOSHA* VITIATION

The concept of *dosha* vitiation is uniquely Ayurvedic. Vitiation is a condition characterized by impairment, imbalance, abnormal excitation, aggravation, excess proliferation, qualitative disturbance, spoiling, and derangement. Vitiation or perturbation of *doshas*, if not checked, heralds the beginning of the disease process. *Doshas* may be vitiated by innumerable factors, but the most common include diet, season, lifestyle and behavior, age, and psychological stress.

Dosha vitiation refers to *doshas* that are abnormally increased and / or qualitatively deranged. The state of abnormally low *doshas* (*dosha kshaya*) is uncommon. The most prevalent lowered *dosha* finding is that related to low *Agni*, a form of lowered *Pitta*. This issue will be elaborated upon in the treatment sections. Lowered *Vata* may suggest insufficient *Prana Vata* or *Apana Vata* and produce symptoms of fatigue or insomnia. Lowered *Kapha* may be related to states of inordinate emaciation and to the wasting diseases. The treatments for lowered *doshas* are usually dietary, and may include appropriate herbs.

Dosha Vitiation Due to Diet

Dosha vitiation is often caused by dietary factors. This type of vitiation may be the most common and significant factor that engenders doshic imbalances. When foods that are not suitable for a specific constitutional type are eaten, they will cause a disturbance in the predominant *dosha* or *doshas* in that *prakruti*. A diet such as this is defined as one having a similar composition, both of the primary Elements and of the specific *doshas*, to that of the individual's *dosha* dominance, the *prakruti*. Examples of this are the following:

1. *Vata* predominant *prakrutis* are exacerbated by foods that increase *Vata* such as beans, raw vegetables, mushrooms, soda, dry breakfast cereals, popcorn, and carbonated beverages, for example. Foods and other dietary substances with tastes that are pungent, bitter, and astringent will increase *Vata*. Dietary habits such as fasting and taking more food before the previous meal has been digested increase *Vata*. In the already *Vata*-dominant *prakruti*, these foods will further increase *Vata* and cause *Vata* vitiation.

2. *Pitta* predominant *prakrutis* are exacerbated by foods that increase *Pitta,* such as salt, nuts, hot vegetables (peppers, onions, tomatoes), alcohol, sour fruits (oranges), vinegar, and very hot spices (red pepper). Foods that have pungent, sour, and salty taste components increase *Pitta.*
3. *Kapha* predominant *prakrutis* are exacerbated by foods that increase *Kapha* such as yogurt, cheese, ice cream, nuts, red meats, oils, cold drinks, and sweets. Foods with predominantly sweet, sour, and salty tastes increase *Kapha.*

Dosha Vitiation Due to Age

As has been described previously, the season of a person's life brings with it a natural dominance of one of the three *doshas. Kapha* predominates from birth through adolescence (*bala*); *Pitta* predominates in adolescence until about age 55 (*madhya*); *Vata* gradually predominates thereafter (*vriddha*). The dominance of a *dosha* according to one's age contributes to an increased susceptibility to that particular *dosha*'s disease tendency. Although this, by itself, is not abnormal, it does predispose to an increased susceptibility to doshic vitiation when other factors such as diet, lifestyle, behavior, and climate contribute their influence.

Dosha Vitiation Due to Season

The normal seasonal fluctuation of the *doshas* has been discussed. This factor, as that of chronological age, does contribute to doshic vitiation. In general, *Pitta* is most increased in the summer and in any hot climate or environmental condition. *Vata* is increased in dry, cold, windy environments such as are found in the fall season. The fall season tends to exert the most severe stress on all the *doshas* in all *prakruti* types. *Kapha* increases when environmental factors include cold, damp, and dark conditions. As with the doshic increases that accompany age, those that set in with changing climatic conditions exert a real influence, but that influence can be considered only partial in its impact. *Doshas* are most disturbed when an array of multiple influences, especially over a significant period, affect them. Diet and season are the most intense sources of doshic provocation.

Dosha Vitiation Due to Lifestyle and Behavior

Lifestyle encompasses those activities of daily living that include such things as sleep patterns, personal hygiene, eating habits, exercise routines, job and career activity, and recreational preferences to name just a few. Each of the three *doshas* is sensitive to a particular type of activity. The following is a representative sampling of behaviors that cause specific *doshas* to become vitiated or increased.

1. *Vata*. Any excess physical activity increases *Vata*. Other excess activities include excess talking and excess traveling, especially because of the jerks and agitation that movement causes. Insofar as sleep goes, *Vata* is increased when one remains awake at night past about 10 P.M. Another concept unique to Ayurveda is that of the *Vega dharana* or the 13 natural urges. They consist of eating, drinking, vomiting, belching, inhalation, yawning, sneezing, urinating, defecating, passing flatus, ejaculation, crying, and sleeping. They are all controlled by the various subdoshas of *Vata*. When any of these natural urges is suppressed, obstructed, or impaired, its complement of *Vata dosha* then becomes vitiated. This vitiation of *Vata* has many imbalancing consequences. One of the most significant is that of the additional vitiation of the specific channel system (*srota*) involved. This vitiation of a particular *srota* causes impaired functioning that may take the form of a reversal of the proper flow (*pratiloma*), a blockage of flow (*srotorhodha*), or a flow outside of the channel and into an inappropriate tissue site (*vimarga gamana*). These abnormal channel impingements create a potential for the disease process to set in.

2. *Pitta dosha* may become vitiated by excessive exposure to heat whether it is climatic or produced by situations such as radiation, machines, saunas, steam baths, fires, tanning booths, etc. Competitive activities, mental or physical, whether in sports or in the job setting contribute to *Pitta* exacerbation.

3. *Kapha dosha* is increased by lifestyles that are slow, sluggish, sedentary, and inordinately inactive. *Kapha* is also increased by excessive sleep, especially during the morning hours and during the daytime.

Dosha Vitiation Due to Psychological Factors

The psychological sphere has cognitive and emotional dimensions. This domain is complex and only a brief outline of pertinent factors will be described. Any rajasic (turbulent) or tamasic (dulling) stimuli will elicit *dosha* vitiation. Any stress may contribute to doshic imbalance. A vicious cycle is set up since when a stressor increases a particular *dosha* then that vitiated *dosha* tends to attract or elicit further stimulation by the original event that triggered it. The following are essential psychological triggers of specific *dosha* vitiations:

1. *Vata* undergoes disruptive excitation when the following are experienced: anxiety, fear, ambivalence, insecurity, impulsivity, hyperactivity, agitation, mania, mood lability, inattentiveness, loquaciousness, inordinate excitability, fear of self-harm, drug addiction, sexual perversion, sexual excess, and psychosis.
2. *Pitta* is vitiated when the following are experienced: anger, aggression, competition, irritability, and controlling, manipulative, and dominating behaviors; also included are envy, pride, narcissism, lustful desire, hate, violence, destructiveness, and criminality.
3. *Kapha* tends to become vitiated when the following are present: greed, inordinate attachment, avaricious lust, rigid materialism, clinging dependency, hedonism, depressions with psychomotor retardation, apathy, inertia, and sloth.

Impairment of *Agni*, the Digestive Fire

Agni, as it exists in the form of the digestive fire or the *Jatharagni*, is one of the most fundamental concepts in Ayurveda. The health or illness of the individual is almost entirely identified with the state of the *Agni*. The digestive fire is the essential transformative force that facilitates proper digestion, absorption, and assimilation of nutrients. *Agni* not only refers to the gastrointestinal digestive processes, but also extends to include the digestion, so to speak, of all psychological experience. *Agni* and metabolic transformations, therefore, take place in the gastrointestinal tract, in the liver, and at the tissue and cellular level throughout the entire body including the brain. *Agni* thus exerts its transformative power in the psychological sphere as well.

According to Ayurveda, *Agni* becomes impaired when the *doshas* become vitiated. Although this includes the *tridosha* (three-*dosha*) group of *Vata, Pitta,* and *Kapha,* the vitiation of *Vata* and of *Kapha* are the conditions that most often impair the digestive fire. *Kapha* excess creates conditions that are cold, damp, and heavy and so contribute to dousing the digestive fire. *Vata* has qualities of cold, exuberant agitation, and mobility that can blow out the flame of the digestive fire. When the digestive fire becomes dulled (*Agnimandya*), all metabolic processes begin to become dysfunctional. Some of the common dietary and lifestyle causes of *Agnimandya* are the following:

1. Overuse of cold foods and liquids
2. Overeating or undereating (i.e., excessive fasting)
3. Heavy foods
4. Meat
5. Eating before the previous meal has been digested
6. Incorrect food combinations
7. Dietary factors such as quality of food, food preparation, *prakruti* incompatible foods, chronological and seasonal specifications for proper foods
8. Suppression of the 13 natural urges
9. Poor sleep patterns
10. Motoric overactivity or underactivity
11. Psychological stressors

The above listing is not exhaustive. It reflects, in part, the previously mentioned factors that contribute to the vitiation of the *doshas*. All doshic vitiation tends to create conditions that impair the *Agni*. When the *Agni* is impaired for a significant period, the toxic metabolic product, *Ama,* is produced. The vitiated *doshas,* along with *Ama,* launch the potential disease process.

Ama

Ama is the Sanskrit word that comes from the root *am* meaning "to harm or to weaken." *Ama* constitutes a diverse group of toxic substances that includes internal metabolic and cellular waste products as well as pollutants and other toxins from the environment that enter the body. The phenomena of free radicals and free radical damaged cellular and tissue debris is included in this idea. The traditional Ayurvedic concept of *Ama* emphasizes the role of seriously impaired *Agni* and its inability to normally digest and metabolize ingested food. The portion of food that cannot be properly digested is considered to be in a "raw" state. This raw, undigested material then stagnates and transforms into a toxic mass of impurities still contained within the gastrointestinal tract. The resulting *Ama* is carried by vitiated *doshas* into the tissue channels of circulation and travels peripherally outside of the gastrointestinal tract. Although *Ama* is propelled by *Vata* to travel in the channels of circulation, its erratic movements are accompanied by a sluggish quality primarily due to the sticky and adhering nature of the *Ama* itself.

Samprapti: Pathogenesis Proper

Samprapti is the heart of the Ayurvedic conceptualization of the development of the disease process. It has been formulated over thousands of years, and remains the group of basic propositions that reflect the Ayurvedic concept of pathogenesis. In its view of ill health, Ayurveda places greater emphasis on the dynamic processes leading up to the manifestation of the disease rather than on the disease itself, as a discrete entity. This view of pathology, therefore, is a more dynamic rather than static one. As has been described previously, the triggers for disease lie in the universal phenomena of *Prajna-aparadha,* which leads to wrong choices in diet, lifestyle, and behavior. Along with these factors, the influence of seasonal variations, and the impact that stressful emotional states and cognitive experience produce together contribute to the vitiation process.

When the *doshas* begin to become increasingly vitiated, the *Agni* becomes impaired and *Ama* is formed. *Ama* then spreads in the channels of circulation and eventually forms significant blockages in weakened channels and tissues. This obstructive process produces the manifestations of disease.

Samprapti, also known as *Shat Kriyakala,* connotes the six physiological states and times during which the disease process develops. The six stages are the following.

1. *Sanchaya,* Accumulation
2. *Prakopa,* Aggravation
3. *Prasara,* Spread
4. *Sthana Samshraya,* Localization
5. *Vyakti,* Manifestation
6. *Bheda,* Differentiation

Sanchaya: Preclinical Stage 1

Sanchaya is the gradual accumulation of a vitiated *dosha* that occurs in that specific *dosha*'s home site within the gastrointestinal tract. This site of origin is called *udbhava sthana.* When vitiated, *Vata* accumulates in the colon; *Pitta* accumulates in the small intestine; and *Kapha* accumulates in the stomach. Signs and symptoms at this early preclinical stage are vague and subtle. *Vata* vitiation may appear as gas, constipation, or the psychological experience of anxiety or fear. *Pitta* vitiation may appear as the sensation of mild heat or burning with a bitter taste in the mouth. *Kapha* vitiation may appear as nausea and the feeling of heaviness. As the body attempts to correct these beginning imbalances, the individual instinctively begins to crave foods and conditions that are opposite to the qualities of the accumulating *doshas.* This is the body's initial and instinctive attempt to restore balance.

Prakopa: Preclinical Stage 2

Prakopa is the continued increase of the vitiated *doshas,* in their own site of origin, to the point of maximal quantity. The *dosha* now is aggravated and "rageful." Signs and symptoms are still vague, but take on a more intense character. *Vata* aggravation may appear as pain, spasm, and abdominal distension. *Pitta* aggravation may appear as acid regurgitation, thirst, and a sour taste in the mouth. *Kapha* aggravation may appear as the loss of appetite, as excess salivation, and as fatigue and lethargy with a need to sleep during the day. As *Vata, Pitta,* and *Kapha* rise to almost maximal intensity, each of them contributes to further diminish the power of *Agni.* The overall metabolic processes therefore decrease. As this occurs, food cannot be transformed properly and completely into healthy, assimilable nutrients, and, therefore, *Ama* formation begins.

Prasara: Preclinical Stage 3

Prasara is the overflow and spread of the maximally elevated *doshas*. They, along with *Ama,* flow out of their respective sites in the gastrointestinal tract, and go into the blood and plasma channels to spread into more peripheral body sites. The seriously aggravated *Vata,* in this condition, takes a wild and explosive course (*prakupita*) that is improper and contrary to a normal healthy flow. Signs and symptoms become more intense although they remain in a preclinical state and are not disease specific. The spreading of *Vata* may appear as joint stiffness, backache, spasm, cough, and the sensation of fullness accompanied by bowel sounds. The spread of *Pitta* may show as diarrhea, bilious vomiting, gingivitis, or pulling and burning sensations. The spreading *Kapha* may be signaled by a low-grade fever, no appetite, and lethargy. These symptoms continue to manifest as vague and ambiguous signs of general malaise.

According to Ayurveda, when the vitiated *doshas* begin to spread, they follow one or more of three distinct pathways (*margas*). Their flow in the channels of circulation is usually away from the center of the body toward the more peripheral, dense, and compact body structures. This outward flow has more disease-producing potential since the vitiated *doshas* are mixed with toxic *Ama* and have a predilection to settle in weakened or damaged tissues. The three disease paths or tracts are:

1. *Antharmarga,* the Inner Gastrointestinal Path. This is also called the *Maha-Srotas,* meaning the great channel, and refers

to the GI tract. Diseases that settle here are easier to treat since their toxins can be eliminated directly through the GI tract, which is the premier method for dispelling vitiated *doshas* and toxins. Many *Kapha*-related diseases take hold in this site.

2. *Bayhamarga,* the Outer Peripheral Path. This is associated with the *shakha* or limbs and includes the paths provided by plasma, blood, and the skin. Diseases that settle here are moderately difficult to treat since they have entered the internal body tissues. *Pitta* diseases, particularly of the blood, follow this path.
3. *Madhyamamarga,* the Central Path. This is composed of the paths to the vital organs and includes the brain, the heart, the kidneys, and five tissues: muscle, fat, bone, marrow/nerve, and reproductive. Disease in these areas is considered most serious and very difficult to treat. It includes chronic and degenerative diseases such as arthritis and cancer, for example. *Vata*-type diseases are most prominent in these areas.

Sthana-Samshraya: Clinical Stage 4

Sthana-samshraya means site of deposition and this clinical stage of pathogenesis is the stage of the relocation of the spreading vitiated *doshas* and *Ama* into a circumscribed area that has already been weakened or damaged in the past. This localization process is considered one of the most critical events in the course of disease formation. It heralds the birth of what may become the final disease condition. Until this event occurs, the pathogenic process has been preclinical, relatively weaker, and accompanied by vague and less definitive symptomatology, and, as well, is more easily treatable.

In this localization phase, the important role of the tissues and the channels in pathogenesis emerges. In the body over time, various events have produced both physical and psychological traumas in the tissues, the organs, and the channels. Causes of weakened or deformed channels, for example, include any or all of the following factors: genetic, congenital, deformity from past disease, external trauma, accidents, poisons, environmental pollutants, and diet and lifestyle practices contrary to one's *prakruti* requirements. Impairment or damage to the channels is exceedingly critical insofar as this constitutes one of the most significant weakened areas that may act like an attractor and as a potential reservoir for the *Ama*-laden vitiated *doshas*. These susceptible areas of devitalization are referred to as *kervaigunya* or weak spots. These weak spots may result from constitutional endowment or from damage by trauma, infection, improper diet, or lifestyle over time. The vitiated tissue, themselves, are called *dusha,* also spelled *doosha* or *dushya.* When the vitiated *Ama*-laden *doshas* find and locate in these *dusha,* this pathogenic merging is called *dosha-dusha sammurchanna.*

Sammurchanna is a pathological amalgamation that produces a new substance that has a qualitatively distinct pathogenic character. This *sammurchanna* causes an overwhelming obstruction within the channels that it attacks, and produces the phenomenon of *srotorhodha* or channel obstruction. This event heralds the actual birth of the disease. Impaired flow through any of the innumerable channels of circulation produces an overall impairment of the individual's quality of life. This is felt in symptoms of malaise and dysphoria, and in premonitory signs of impending poor health.

One of the most important therapeutic concepts contained in the understanding of this stage of disease is the overwhelming emphasis on the aberrant or vitiated tissue that is able to attract, receive, and hold the *Ama*-laden vitiated *doshas* in the disease process. Disease is only possible when tissue is devitalized. This takes into serious account the concept of resistance to disease and immunity. Only when resistance and immunity are lowered, that is, when there is sufficient tissue vitiation, will disease take hold. The concept of "germs" that includes invading bacteria, viruses, and other pathogens was known in ancient times and is referred to by the Sanskrit word *krimi* in the *Rig-Veda,* the *Charaka,* and the *Sushruta Samhita* medical texts. While attention was given to these pathogens, the major emphasis in preventing and treating disease was placed on the condition of the tissues. Treatments were aimed at strengthening, restoring, and healing the tissues in order to make them unreceptive and resistant to pathogens. This emphasis on tissue health included not only nourishment and restoration, but went beyond and addressed issues of rejuvenation.

Channel obstruction produces a relatively more specific group of prodromal signs and symptoms called *Purva Rupa*. These premonitory signals appear before the actual distinct manifestations of a disease. They can provide clues to impending disease consolidation, especially because the signs and symptoms are now more fixed in location and not merely in the process of wandering.

An important aspect of this stage in the pathogenic process consists of its organizing capacity. A disease process differentiates and takes on a particular identity specifically because of its channel, organ, or tissue involvement. The same *dosha* or *doshas* may produce different types of diseases. The doshic component, therefore, is nonspecific although necessary. The channel component is the most critical factor in determining the identity of a particular disease. Channels of circulation are an intrinsic part of the matrix of every bodily substance. Any impairment of channel structure or functioning affects not only the channel, itself, but also the tissues, organs, etc., that it manages in terms of nutrition and removal of wastes.

Vyakti: Clinical Stage 5

Vyakti is the clinical stage of the actual manifestation of the disease. At this point, the full display of a particular disease makes its appearance. The actual signs and symptoms of a disease are called *Rupa*. The site of manifestation where a disease displays its signs and symptoms is called the *adhisthana*.

The range of categories of *Rupa* includes the following:

1. *Samanya lakshana*, general characteristics
2. *Visista*, specific and cardinal characteristics
3. Invariable signs and symptoms
4. *Upadrava*, complications
5. *Aristha*, prognosis

Bheda: Clinical Stage 6

The last stage of *Samprapti* is *Bheda,* the stage of differentiation. It is here that the manifestation of a disease becomes consolidated and most specific. This differentiation process usually proceeds along the lines of the predominant *dosha* and its tissue involvement. Disease complications also develop from this stage.

TYPES OF *SAMPRAPTI*

Samprapti may be categorized in two ways. The first is according to the type and number of *doshas* involved. When only one *dosha* is involved, the *samprapti* is called *nanatmaja.* When two different *doshas* are involved, the *samprapti* is termed *samanyaja.* When all three *doshas* participate, the disease process is referred to as *sannipatta.* Ayurveda has also given an estimation of the number of different diseases for each *dosha* predominance. There are 80 *Vata*-predominant diseases, 40 *Pitta*-predominant diseases, and 20 *Kapha*-predominant diseases (see Appendix 2).

The second main classification of *samprapti* is according to the leading features of the predominant *dosha's* qualities or attributes. This assessment is based on the appearance of the various attributes that are specifically related to the particular *dosha* involved. An example of this would be differentiating the disease of arthritis into either a *Vata* arthritis (with symptoms and signs of pain, coldness, stiffness, etc.), a *Pitta* arthritis (with signs and symptoms of burning pain, red and hot joints, etc.), or a *Kapha* arthritis (with signs and symptoms of swelling, edema, etc.). *Vata* attributes that would be outstanding here are cold, hard, and rough; *Pitta* attributes would be hot and sharp; and *Kapha* attributes would be cold, damp, heavy, and static.

CHAPTER 7

HEALTH AND THE DISEASE PROCESS. II

THE AYURVEDIC CONCEPT OF DISEASE

The Ayurvedic concept of disease is based on the abnormal functioning of the *doshas,* and is manifest in the imbalanced state of the *prakruti* (constitutional type) called the *vikruti* (imbalanced constitution). The presence of the *vikruti* connotes an impairment of *Agni* or the digestive fire, an accumulation of *Ama* or toxic impurities, vitiated *doshas,* and a dysfunction of the *dhatus* (tissues), *malas* (wastes), and *Manas* (mental and emotional functioning). The patient feels characteristic symptoms, and the practitioner can ascertain signs of the disease. *Purva rupa* refers to that group of prodromal signs and symptoms that precede the actual manifestation of the disease. It is at this preclinical juncture, before disease sets in, that Ayurvedic medicine is able to detect an imbalance and intervene to prevent the progression toward disease eruption. *Rupa* refers to the cluster of signs and symptoms that accompany the full manifestation of the disease. For disease to actually take hold, not only do the *doshas* need to be in a state of vitiation but localized pathology, specifically in deep tissue areas, needs to be present and acted upon by the vitiated *doshas.* In effect, disease manifests in a wide variety of discrete disorders as well as in broader syndrome complexes. The complex of physical pain and mental suffering, however, constitutes the ultimate disease condition and its incarnations are manifold.

ETIOLOGICAL FACTORS CAUSING DISEASE: *NIDANA*

The term *Nidana* refers to etiology and to diagnosis. It is the broadest umbrella under which the spectrum of disease causing factors is subsumed. *Nidana* is the term given to an etiological factor usually when it causes the full development of the disease process; as such, these causes are determined retrospectively, at times. As has been discussed previously, three fundamental causes are considered the universal reasons for any disease to occur. They are *Prajna-aparadha* (errors in wisdom), *Asatmyendriyartha samyoga* (inappropriate contact between the sense organs and their objects), and *Kala-Parinama* (effects of time). These three determinants involve axiomatic propositions and rest heavily on theoretical foundations. While these are at the base of all disease manifestations, additional causes may be regarded as particular variables. Classification of these variables includes aspects of the multiple causative factors of disease considered from varying perspectives such as location, timing, insidiousness, external factors, internal contributory processes, etc. A discussion of some of the various classifications will follow.

SPECTRUM OF TERMS DENOTING ETIOLOGY

The commonly used terms describing the more concrete precipitants of disease are *hetu* and *karana*. Other terms with differing connotations are the following. The cause of a disease that specifies its path and spread is called *ayatana*. A cause that shows a close relationship to effect is called *pratyaya*. The root cause of a disease is referred to as *mula*; and the site or origin of a disease is called *yoni*. The term *karta* refers to that which creates a disease; for example, the *doshas* are considered the creators of disease. *Utthana* and *samutthana* are causative factors that stimulate dormant *doshas*, activate and vitiate them. Endogenous causes are termed *nija*; exogenous causes are termed *agantu*.

As far as strength and time of onset, disease causes fall into four categories:

1. *Sannikrushta* refers to causes that produce disease early on and bypass the accumulation phase of *samprapti*. The *doshas*

suddenly become aggravated in intensity and produce symptoms. Examples of this are: exposure to cold producing sudden attacks of sinusitis; allergens producing sudden allergic reactions; or damp spring weather triggering an asthmatic attack.

2. *Viprakrushta* refers to causative factors of longer duration that produce delayed results. Examples include chronic smoking leading to emphysema, and chronic alcohol use leading to hepatic impairment.
3. *Vyabhichari* refers to very feeble causes that are not strong enough to produce disease unless other intensifying factors such as chronic duration accompany them.
4. *Pradhanik* refers to causes that are fulminating and produce immediate and serious, life threatening disease. Examples include accidents, trauma, strong toxins, poisons, and some microbial causes.

Another classification system groups variations of causative factors in the following three ways.

1. *Utpadaka* refers to causes that directly vitiate the *doshas*. This refers most specifically to dietary provocations.
2. *Vyadhi pratyanika* refers to specific causes for specific diseases. Examples are infectious sexual contact possibly causing HIV and hepatitis; pica causing anemia and allied conditions; and close contact with already infected patients transferring bacteria to cause conjunctivitis.
3. *Ubhaya hetu* refers to causes that include both of the above, i.e., vitiation of *doshas* and disease-causing specificity. An example illustrating this is the chronic use of alcohol that leads to *Pitta dosha* vitiation and subsequently to hepatic impairment and cirrhosis.

An ancient classification system, based on three primary locations of the etiological events that produce the disease, is as follows.

1. *Adhyatmika* refers to causation that originates within the body. It is subdivided into three groups:

(a) *Adhibala*: genetic causes
(b) *Janmaja*: congenital causes
(c) *Dosaja:* vitiated *doshas* as primary causative factors

2. *Adhibhautika* refers to causation coming from external causes such as germs, trauma, and accidents.

3. *Adhidaivika* refers to causes that are considered providential, due to Fate, Karma, and other more esoteric sources.

Some disease categorizations reflect a more general yet dynamic perspective. Accordingly, disease etiology, as *hetu* or *karana,* consists of the following three components:

1. *Nimmitta* refers to the necessary precipitating or hastening causes such as diet, lifestyle, season (*kalabala*), age (*swabhavabala*), and psychological factors.
2. *Samavayi* are the components that are the matrix within which the disease manifests. They would be the *doshas, dhatus, srotas,* etc.
3. *Asamavayi* refers to the interaction of the entire spectrum of components, i.e., *doshas, dhatus, srotas,* etc., which combine and interact to yield the final disease product.

CLASSIFICATION OF DISEASE ACCORDING TO PROGNOSIS

Ayurveda divides diseases into two broad prognostic categories: (1) curable and (2) incurable. Curable diseases are either easily treated or resolve with difficulty. Incurable diseases need either long-term maintenance or they may lead to death.

Curable diseases are termed *sukha sadhya*. Their characteristics include minimal severity, *dosha* and affected tissue being not similar in Elemental composition, the vitiated *dosha* not being part of the patient's *prakruti,* and the vitiated *dosha* not being similar to the current season and climate. The ancient Ayurvedic texts also included the need for the "four essential factors for good treatment" to be present. They are (1) a knowledgeable physician; (2) a caring nurse or attendant; (3) proper medicine; and (4) a compliant patient.

Difficult to cure diseases are more severe, have *dosha* and affected tissue of similar Elemental composition, have *doshas* that are part of the patient's predominant *prakruti,* and occur in a season and climate that exacerbates the already affected *doshas*. *Vata*-dominant diseases are considered the most difficult since *Vata dosha* tends to travel and penetrate into deeper tissues, i.e., bone, nerves, reproductive, and include aspects of psychological dysfunction. *Kapha* diseases are considered most amenable to treatment, and *Pitta* diseases fall in between as far as severity and prognosis are concerned.

Palliable diseases termed *yappa* require long-term maintenance. They are characterized by the involvement of two or more *doshas* simultaneously, by involvement of the central vital organ tract where deeper tissues are involved, and may require treatments that involve surgical procedures.

Intractable diseases termed *asadhya* have very poor or morbid prognoses. They are characterized by the involvement of multiple *doshas,* tissues, organs, and the deeper, vital structures of the body.

CLASSIFICATION OF DISEASE ACCORDING TO STAGES OF THE DISEASE PROCESS

The major staging classification of the disease process has been described as the sequence of *dosha* vitiation and pathological interaction with the tissue elements, i.e., *samprapti*. In *samprapti* proper, at the fourth stage of localization of vitiated *doshas* and *Ama* merging with vitiated tissues, the condition of the *doshas* and tissues is termed *sama dosha* and *sama dhatu,* respectively. When the *doshas* are therapeutically cleansed of toxins, they are called *nirama doshas*. There is, therefore, a *sama* stage of disease and a *nirama* stage of disease. There are additional descriptive stages. When a disease is relatively new, it is referred to as *nava;* when chronic, as *jeerna*. When the disease is more superficial, it is called *uttana;* when deep, it is termed *gambhira*. Superficial diseases usually affect the plasma and the blood; deep disease affects the muscle, fat, bone, nerve, and reproductive tissues. Two phases of the explicitness of a disease are described: (1) *vega,* when the disease is urged to manifest; and (2) *avega,* when the disease is hidden in the *dhatus* (tissues) by the masking power of *Vata.*

SIGNS AND SYMPTOMS OF THE DISEASE PROCESS

The disease process is a gradual development that begins with vitiated *doshas* and eventually affects all the other body's constituents and functioning. Pain, malaise, and discomfort attend all disease. *Vata dosha*'s involvement is usually essential. Pain due to vitiated *Vata* is characterized as radiating, shifting, shooting, pulsating, and irregular. Pain due to vitiated *Pitta* obstructing *Vata* is felt as burning, cutting, penetrating, intense, and producing heat and redness. Pain due to vitiated *Kapha* obstructing *Vata* is felt as heavy, dull, aching, and throbbing. Pain due to *Ama* obstructing *Vata* usually is felt as dull and very heavy, almost leaden in quality. Signs and symptoms of this evolving imbalanced state, therefore, span a continuum from subclinical to clinical manifestations. A general orientation describing *dosha* vitiation and some specific and clinically decipherable disease syndromes according to channel vitiation will be reviewed.

Indicators of *Vata* Vitiation

The chief clinical manifestation of *Vata* vitiation in the body is pain. Most of the signs and symptoms that *Vata* produces derive from an intensification of its attributes or *gunas. Vata* vitiation tends to create tissue loss (*dhatuksaya*) with tissue porosity and dilatation and atrophy, excess movement, and hypersensitivity. In addition, one may find the following: spasm, tremors (*kampa*), horripilation, numbness, contraction, obstruction associated with atrophy and vasospasm, ptosis, stiffness, constipation, cracking sounds from joints, trembling, dehydration, thirst, rough dry skin, agitation, astringent taste in mouth, and red, black, or brown discolorations (*arunasayava*) of the skin or other tissues. The principal manifestations of *Vata* vitiation in the psychological sphere include anxiety, manic-depression, agitation, hyperactivity, insomnia, and chronic low energy. The strong *Rajasic* (turbulent) components within *Vata* directly contribute to its agitating and disorganizing power in the mental sphere. The intensely driven quality of some psychiatric disorders, i.e., hyperactivity, agitated depression, and bipolar mania, are manifestations of this.

Indicators of *Pitta* Vitiation

The chief clinical manifestation of *Pitta* vitiation in the body is inflammation. Aggravated *Pitta* manifests as burning sensations, redness, increased temperature, sweating, hot, sensitive and oily skin, boils, pus formation, hemorrhagic disorders, necrosis, gangrene, dry mouth and thirst, hyperacidity, pungent, bitter, or sour taste in the mouth, and skin and tissue discolorations of any color other than white or brownish black. Different forms of syncope or fainting may be a sign of *Pitta* aggravation. In the psychological sphere, *Pitta* vitiation may produce moderate insomnia, irritability, anger, inordinate competitiveness, obsessive–compulsive behavior, and states of disorientation as, for example, the intoxicated and inebriated condition. Chronic states of exhaustion may have a strong vitiated *Pitta* component since chronic *Pitta* excesses may tend to "burnout" or begin to damage aspects of the central nervous system including neurotransmitter functioning.

Indicators of *Kapha* Vitiation

The chief clinical manifestations of vitiated *Kapha* in the body include heaviness, edema, swelling, and obstruction. Vitiated *Kapha* also appears as increased mucous production or phlegm, increased salivation, respiratory congestion, cold sensations, torpor, lethargy, inertia, somnolence, impaired and sluggish digestion, itching of the skin, cold and oily skin, hardening of the tissues (i.e., lithiasis, tumor, atheroma), obstruction in the channels due to excesses of blocking substances, white or pale skin color and pallor, and sweet or salty taste in the mouth. In the psychological domain, vitiated *Kapha* is reflected in states of severe dependency and in inordinate attachment behaviors. Severe depressions with psychomotor retardation are reflective of the strong tamasic (dulling) component within *Kapha* when it is exacerbated and displayed in the emotional realm.

Disease Manifestations Due to Channel Vitiation

The *srotas* or channels of circulation constitute an integral network throughout the body coordinating the integrity of its functioning. For any disease to exert some significant systemic impairment, not only the *doshas* but also the *dhatus* or tissues and the *srotas* or tissue channels need to be affected and involved in a pathological interaction. An outline of the channels with some common vitiating factors and some characteristic clinical manifestations of impairment will follow.

Pranavaha Srotas constitutes the respiratory and *Prana* carrying channels. They have an intimate connection to the heart, lungs, brain, and colon. Causes of vitiation include malnutrition, wasting diseases, excessive physical exercise, smoking cigarettes, environmental pollutants, and the suppression of the natural urges (*vega-dharana*). *Vata* vitiation, in particular, adversely affects this channel. Signs and symptoms include any respiratory difficulty such as cough, dyspnea, and asthma; as well as disorders related to energy level and psychological status.

Annavaha Srotas constitutes the entire gastrointestinal tract. Causes of vitiation include impairments of the digestive fire, and improper dietary behavior such as overeating, eating at the wrong times, and eating foods contrary to one's needs. Disturbances include all digestive disorders, appetite dysregulation, vomiting, diarrhea, and constipation.

Ambuvaha Srotas is the water regulatory system. Vitiating factors include exposure to excess heat, alcohol, and salt, dehydration, *Ama* buildup, and the experience of inordinate fear.

Signs of disorder include inordinate thirst, edema, blood glucose dysregulation, and diabetes.

Rasavaha Srotas is the lymphatic or plasma channel. Factors that damage these channels include impaired digestive fire with *Ama* buildup, improper absorption of nutrients, excess food and beverage intake, and inordinate stress. Signs of vitiation include anorexia, premature wrinkling of skin, premature graying of hair, impotence, lymphatic disorders, and fungal infections.

Raktavaha Srotas is the blood circulatory system. Damaging factors include diets with foods and herbs that are too stimulating (*vidahi*) and hot, and by overexposure to intensive environmental heat. Signs of vitiation include all the hematological disorders, skin disorders such as acne and rashes, hypertension, hypotension, arrhythmias, liver and spleen disorders, and hemorrhagic disorders.

Mamsavaha Srotas includes the muscular and integumentary systems. Vitiations are believed to result from over consumption of foods that are heavy and oily, and by frequent sleeping after meals. Signs of disorder include muscle dysfunction such as excess activity (tremor, spasm), hypoactivity, atony, tissue tears, and tumors.

Medovaha Srotas includes the channels of adipose tissue especially around the kidneys and within the abdominal omental sheaths. Vitiating factors, mainly dietary, include excess intake of foods, especially with a high fat content, excess intake of alcohol, and sleep during the daytime. Signs of disorder include obesity, edema, fatty tumors, hypertension, heart disease, cholesterol and blood lipid disorders, diabetes, and arthritis.

Asthivaha Srotas refers to the skeletal system. Damaging factors include trauma and any food, herb, or physical activity that increases *Vata*. Excessive physical activity to the point of sweating and shortness of breath, i.e., aerobic exercise, running, jogging, and strenuous manual labor normally increase *Vata*. This becomes damaging only over a long period of time if *Vata* is not periodically reduced in order to prevent inordinate cumulative effects. This point emphasizes the Ayurvedic ideal of continually attempting to restore balance to imbalanced states since it is natural to engage in activities that may tend toward excess and subsequent dysfunction. Signs and symptoms include any bone disorders such as osteoporosis, hypertrophy, arthritis, as well as some disorders of hair and nails.

Majjavaha Srotas refers to the nervous system and aspects of the long bones and joints. Damaging factors include trauma, especially the fracture of the long bones, and the ingestion of what Ayurveda considers "incompatible food combinations" (to be discussed later). Psychological trauma is also considered a vitiating factor. Any high *Vata* or high *Pitta* stimuli are particularly traumatic. Manifestations of disturbance include pain in the joints, lack of coordination, paresis or paralysis of muscle, convulsion, coma, multiple sclerosis, central nervous system and peripheral nervous system dysfunction, as well as distinctive abnormalities in sensory perception, especially that of touch and temperature.

Shukravaha Srotas refers to the reproductive system, and this usually indicates the male system. In addition to physical trauma, Ayurveda considers behavioral factors to be vitiating to this system. The range includes excessive and aberrant sexual practices, inordinate suppression of the sexual urge, and trauma from accidents, surgery, or chemotherapy. Close attention is paid to sexual activity because excessive activity is believed to deplete *Ojas* (vigor and immune functioning) that, in turn, increases *Vata* and diminishes longevity. In addition to disorders of impotence and sexual dysfunction, other diseases affecting the immune system such as tuberculosis and AIDS may result.

Svedavaha Srotas is the perspiratory and sebaceous system. Damaging factors include excess physical activity, excess exposure to heat, cold, and wind, ingestion of excessively hot and pungent foods, alcohol intake, as well as psychological factors such as fear and anger. Signs include disorders of perspiration and some skin disorders.

Mutravaha Srotas refers to the urinary system. Vitiating factors include excessive or insufficient intake of fluids, exposure to inordinately hot and dry climates, excess sexual activity, suppression of the urge to micturate, renal diseases, and trauma. Disease is reflected in any urinary disorder including infection, stones, and tumors.

Purishavaha Srotas refers to the excretory system. Vitiating factors include impaired digestive fire, digestive disturbances, and dietary irregularities. Signs of disorder include constipation, diarrhea, colitis, tumors, hemorrhoids, and any other bowel dysfunction.

Artavavaha Srotas refers to the female reproductive system. Vitiating factors are similar to those that vitiate the *Shukravaha Srotas* and include excessive or suppressed sexual activity, improper dietary practices, and emotional factors such as anxiety, fear, and anger. Signs of disorder include premenstrual tension (PMS), dysmenorrhea, amenorrhea, and menorrhagia.

Stanyavaha Srotas is the female lactation system. The breasts and nipples are the main sites. Vitiating factors are considered to include suppression of breast milk by not breastfeeding and, on the other hand, by excessive breastfeeding. Disorders are thought to include conditions of deficient or excessive lactation, and breast dysfunction such as pain, cysts, and tumors.

Manovaha Srotas refers to the channels that are associated with mental and emotional functioning. Vitiating factors include emotional trauma, illicit substance use, excessive sensory input, and other factors that reflect *vatagenic* (*Vata* provoking) stimuli. Manifestations of disorder include the spectrum of psychological disorders. *Vata* disorders manifest as anxiety, fear, and bipolar conditions. *Pitta* disorders manifest as intense anger, irritability, hostility, and aggressive symptoms. *Kapha* disorders manifest as inordinate dependency and attachment problems, and as retarded depressions.

DIAGNOSTIC EXAMINATION OF THE DISEASE: *ROGA PARIKSHA*

The comprehensive diagnostic assessment requires that the disease itself be examined using a variety of parameters. There are five standard approaches that classical Ayurveda uses to ascertain the major components associated with disease. They include an examination of the following.

1. *Nidana,* causative factors
2. *Purva Rupa,* prodromal symptoms
3. *Rupa,* actual signs and symptoms
4. *Upashaya,* suitability of the means of alleviation. This method consists of the use of exploratory interventions used when the more exact nature of a disease is unclear. *Upashaya* procedures involve therapeutic trials of a variety of treatments to assess whether alleviation of the problem or an exacerbation of it results.
5. *Samprapti,* pathogenesis

DIAGNOSTIC EVALUATION OF THE PATIENT

Diagnosis, in Ayurvedic medicine, is evaluation of the patient's *prakruti* and *vikruti* as a prelude to employing strategies to balance and restore optimal functioning to the *doshas.* Disease is viewed as any disorder disrupting the proper balance of the *doshas.* The diagnostic assessment delineates the basic *prakruti* and what should be the proper functioning of each *dosha,* alone and in interaction with the body's other *doshas.* In addition, this assessment evaluates the quality of the tissues, channels, organs, wastes, and *Manas.*

Diagnostic evaluation is a comprehensive assessment of the patient using a variety of different techniques. The physician arrives at his diagnostic and prognostic assessment by relying on three facets contributing to an understanding of the clinical examination. They are the following.

1. *Aptopadesha/Shabda,* authoritative knowledge. This information derives from two sources. One is the body of theoretical and clinical information found in the literature of Ayurveda, and in the teachings of recognized Ayurvedic physicians. The

other involves the historical data gathered by the clinical interview. These include reports from the patient (*prashna pariksha*), his family, and any other past medical and psychosocial history.

2. *Pratyaksha,* use of the physician's five senses. This is the clinical examination using the physician's direct perception. The functioning of the five senses or *jnanendriyas* are highly regarded in the Ayurvedic system. As such, they have a critically important role to play in diagnostic assessments. The physician becomes, as it were, an instrument, and his five sensory faculties are used as precision tools to explore the patient's presentation.

   Examination using the ear or sense of hearing listens not only to the patient's voice but also to sounds coming from joints, intestines, lungs, etc. The physician also uses supplemental devices such as the stethoscope to hear cardiac and respiratory sounds. Examination with the eye or inspection is a visual survey of appearance, demeanor, and functioning. Examination using the nose or sense of smell can detect an irregularity in body odor, and give an indication of personal hygiene. Examination by touch or palpation supplies data about skin temperature, turgor, abdominal and thoracic organs, and tenderness or sensitivity to pain. Pulse diagnosis is included here (Lad, 1996). Examination by using the sense of taste usually is not done in current times.
3. *Anumana,* reasoning based on inference. This involves the analytic and synthetic interpretation of all the data gathered from the physician's theoretical knowledge and the patient's clinical presentation. This process produces a diagnosis, prognosis, and suggests a treatment plan.

DIAGNOSTIC PROCEDURES IN THE CLINICAL EXAMINATION

Ayurveda has formalized the clinical examination and suggested a systematic strategy for surveying important aspects of the patient's strengths and weaknesses. There are two major groups of methodology. They are the following.

***Dashavidha Pariksha*, The Tenfold Examination**

Charaka has advocated a method that encompasses a comprehensive clinical review incorporating the major areas that are of significance to the Ayurvedic system. They are:

1. *Prakruti*, body constitution
2. *Vikruti*, doshic imbalances
3. *Sara*, tissue quality. This is a survey and estimation of the excellence or optimal quality of each of the seven body tissue systems.
4. *Samhanana*, body conformation. This refers to an assessment of the body build or compactness of the body as a whole. It includes an estimation of symmetry, proportion, nutritional status, general functioning, and movement.
5. *Anguli pramana*, body proportion measurement. This refers to an ancient Ayurvedic concept using mathematical formulas with Ayurvedic measurements called "finger units" to assess the proportions of the body and limbs.
6. *Satyma* or wholesomeness. This represents the patient's adaptability to healthy and optimal diet, herbs, climate, and lifestyle. *Satyma* assesses the patient's natural inclination to gravitate toward and incorporate *prakruti* compatible, sattvic food choices and behaviors.
7. *Manas prakruti*, psychological constitution. This is an evaluation of the proportions of the *Maha gunas, Sattva, Rajas*, and *Tamas*, that are constitutionally inherent, motivate the patient, and guide his lifestyle choices.
8. *Agni* or *Ahara shakti*, digestive fire. This refers to estimating the power of digestive functioning as a result of the quality of the patient's *Agni*.
9. *Vyayama shakti*, capacity for exercise and energy level. This involves an assessment of the general state of energy and endurance, especially concerning physical activity.
10. *Vaya*, age. The actual chronological age of the patient is compared to his current functional level of health and vitality.

In addition, the doshic stage of life, i.e., early life (*bala*) *Kapha* predominance, midlife (*madhya*) *Pitta* predominance, and older age (*vriddha*) *Vata* predominance, is taken into account.

Ashtavidha Pariksha: The Eightfold Examination

This is a more current and succinct method that particularly takes into account pulse diagnosis. Since a working knowledge of these procedures requires formal training and actual clinical experience, only a brief but representative description of each will follow.

1. *Nadi Pariksha,* pulse diagnosis. Ayurvedic pulse diagnosis is different from Western pulse assessments. *Nadi* here refers to the arterial pulse; usually the radial pulse is measured. The physician uses three fingers simultaneously. The index finger is placed over the radial artery closest to the wrist; this area reflects the *Vata* aspect of the pulse. Its sensory impression suggests a characteristic movement (*gati*) resembling that of a snake (*Sarpagati*). When *Vata* is vitiated, the *Vata* pulse is irregular, unsteady, and difficult to detect. It has an insubstantial quality to it. The *Vata* pulse has a low volume and tension, is subtle, and has the weakest or "emptiest" force behind it. Its snakelike character gives it a feel that is thready, narrow, and thin. It tends to be the fastest pulse of the three.

The middle finger is positioned proximal to the index finger and is over the *Pitta* aspect of the pulse. Its sensory impression suggests the leaping movements of a frog (*Mandukagati*). When aspects of *Pitta* are vitiated, the pulse has qualities that are warm, rapid, and thin. It is the strongest pulse and has the highest amplitude which noticeably drops after each beat. Its froglike character gives a feel that is wiry, taut, tight, jumping and bounding in quality.

The ring finger is placed next to the middle finger in the direction of the elbow. This is the *Kapha* aspect of the pulse, and it has the characteristic movement of a swan (*Hamsagati*). When vitiated, this pulse is steady, cold, thick, full, and substantial. Its volume and rhythm are balanced and full. The swan and elephantlike character gives the *Kapha* pulse qualities that are slow, wide, broad, large, deep, rolling, graceful, and slippery.

Pulse rate (*spandana sankhya*) is approximately 80 to 100 beats per minute for *Vata*, 65 to 80 for *Pitta*, and around 70 and lower for *Kapha*. The most accurate pulse reading occurs first in the early morning before food and exertion. The physician uses the right hand and takes the pulse on the right hand of a male and on the left hand of a female. Pulse diagnosis requires a high level of diagnostic sophistication and requires years of training to obtain proficiency. Nuances of the *prakruti* that include information about the subdoshas are discernible.

2. *Jihva Pariksha,* tongue diagnosis. The size, color, coating, and moisture of the tongue are inspected. Small size, pale color, brown or black coating, and dryness indicate *Vata*. Average size, reddish color, yellow coating, and a tendency to dryness indicate *Pitta*. A large tongue that is pale with a moist and whitish coating indicates *Kapha*.
3. *Drika Pariksha,* eye diagnosis. *Vata* signs are dryness and possible tics or twitches. *Pitta* signs are redness and irritation. *Kapha* signs show as watery eyes.
4. *Sparsa Pariksha,* touch diagnosis. This includes detecting the temperature of the skin and abdominal palpation.
5. *Shabda Pariksha,* voice diagnosis. The *Vata* voice is variable in tone and tends to be breathy and relatively indistinct. The *Pitta* voice is sharp, clear, and precise. The *Kapha* voice has a deep tone and is soft and melodious.
6. *Akriti Pariksha,* general appearance diagnosis. This is an important part of the examination and gives both specific and general information concerning the patient's physical body and psychological demeanor. As applies to the other elements of the clinical examination, a further elaboration of technique is beyond the scope of the present work.
7. *Mutra Pariksha,* urine diagnosis. Ayurvedic medicine uses a unique method in assessing the condition of the patient by examining the urine using the addition of drops of oil to the surface. The behavior of the oil droplets is associated with the doshic quality, the severity, and the prognosis of the disease.

8. *Purisha Pariksha,* feces diagnosis. Stool samples are examined for appearance, color, odor, and behavior when placed in a small amount of water. These data reflect the state of the *Agni,* the *doshas,* and the presence of *Ama.*

COMPLEXITY OF THE DISEASE PROCESS AND OF DIAGNOSIS

Ayurveda acknowledges the complexity of the disease process and the difficulty in arriving at an accurate diagnosis. Charaka recognized the intricacies and variations of morphology and the dynamic nature of physiological and metabolic processes from the cellular through the tissue, organ, and system level over 2,000 years ago. Concerning this he says:

> When classified according to cause, pain, color, site, form, and nomenclature, the number of diseases becomes really countless. A physician need not be ashamed if he is not able to name all diseases, as there can be no definite standardization for all diseases. The same provoked *dosha* may produce a variety of diseases according to diversity of causes and to location. Therefore, treatment should be initiated after diagnosing the nature of the disease (with the vitiated *dosha* and *dushya*), and any special causative factors. (*Charaka Samhita,* Sutra Sthana 18.42–44)

CHAPTER 8

NUTRITION AND DIET IN AYURVEDA

THE CONCEPT OF NUTRITION IN AYURVEDA: THEORETICAL CONSIDERATIONS

The concept of nutrition (*annapanavidhi*) in Ayurveda, like other fundamental Ayurvedic propositions, is thousands of years old (Mukerjee, 1974). It is based on empirical evidence derived from health maintenance practices and disease interventions using dietary and adjunctive herbal and mineral preparations. Nutrition as dietetics and food intake (*ahara*) is considered one of the three main pillars upon which the life of the body is supported. The other two pillars are sleep and regulation of proper sexual functioning.

Dravyaguna Shastra (Sharma, 1976), the science of the attributes and actions of substances on the body when taken internally, is the term for the ancient system formalized to explain the nutritive and pharmacological effects of both food and medicine. *Dravyaguna Shastra* constituted a rational attempt at standardization and grew out of the empirical work of practitioners throughout the centuries. Any substance that can be ingested, therefore, such as food, liquids, herbs, minerals, etc., is governed by the principles established by this system of physiological and pharmacological action. In Ayurveda, this concept is broadened to include the range of sensory experience as well as motor activity which is believed to be ingested and taken into the mental faculties as mental nourishment and thereby contributes to the overall nutrition of the individual.

Dravyaguna Shastra, Ayurveda's Materia Medica, is a rational system that outlines the cellular and physiological mechanisms concerned with the pharmacokinetic and pharmacodynamic processes of the body after substances are ingested. The Sanskrit term *dravya* refers to a fundamental concept that connotes any particular substance with emphasis on its material constitution. *Guna* refers to the attributes or qualities of a substance. *Shastra* refers to a methodical instruction system (a textbook). Other essential concepts in this system include the idea of *karma,* the action and consequences of a substance; *samanya,* the therapeutic principle of "like increasing like"; and *vishesha,* the therapeutic principle of "opposites cure or balance each other." The last major proposition in this pharmacological perspective is contained in the Sanskrit term *samavaya,* which refers to an overriding principle of interactive unification. This means that one substance (*dravya*) contains within itself an inseparable linkage to its inherent qualities (*gunas*) and their necessary actions and effects (*karma*).

The boundaries of meaning and usage in Ayurveda among such diverse categories as those that encompass foods, herbs, drugs, as well as the sensory and motor experience of lifestyle and behavior are marginal and exceedingly porous. Dietary substances refer to those ingested materials that give energy to bodily processes, replenish utilized bodily components, and provide overall nutrition and nourishment. Foods are characterized by an emphasis on *rasa* (taste), greater quantitative intake, and replenishment of the Elements (Ether, Air, Fire, Water, and Earth) in order to maintain doshic balance (*Vata, Pitta,* and *Kapha*). Foods and spices are for daily consumption. Drugs, in the Ayurvedic sense, refer to any ingested medicinal substances such as herbs and minerals that act in a therapeutic manner to induce doshic balance in the presence of significant imbalance, restore vitiated tissues, and alleviate disordered conditions. The therapeutic action of medicinal substances is dominated mostly by the *virya* (potency, energy) of the substance. The *vipaka* (post-digestive effect) is also more important in eliciting a therapeutic effect than the *rasa* (taste). The *prabhava,* a substance's special, unusual, and idiosyncratic action, however, overrides all else. Consequently, this requires consumption of much smaller quantities because of the greater intrinsic therapeutic potency of the substance and its ability to destroy *Ama* (toxins) and pacify vitiated *doshas*. This chapter, then, in covering the principles of Ayurvedic nutrition as it pertains to dietary food intake, also covers the fundamental theoretical principles of *Dravyaguna Shastra*.

THE PROPERTIES OF FOODS, HERBS, AND MINERALS

In Ayurveda, the fundamental properties of foods, herbs, and minerals are conceptually analyzed and understood as consisting of four categories of component parts. They are the following:

1. *Maha gunas*. This consists of the major subtle qualities of *Sattva* (purity), *Rajas* (turbulence), and *Tamas* (inertia) that are contained in a substance. Through experience and the analytic methods of *Dravyaguna Shastra*, each food article and each medicinal substance has been recognized as having a predominance of one of these universal, binding factors. A substance actually evokes a particular *Maha guna* increase in an individual rather than merely containing it apart from human contact.
2. *Gurvadi gunas*. These are the 10 pairs of opposite attributes (hot / cold, heavy / light, oily / dry, stable / mobile, hard / soft, clear / cloudy, rough / smooth, gross / subtle, and liquid / dense) that characterize all materials. Ayurveda considers that virtually every manifestation in the created world can be described using several of these fundamental properties. They impart stylistic form to its substantive Elemental content. These attributes have physical and tangible status as well as having internal pharmacological actions.
3. *Elements*. The five great gross Elements or *Mahabhutanis* are the elemental building blocks of all material substances. These Elements are the chief templates that impart substantive identity to a physical substance. Every substance contains all five Elements, but only one or two Elements predominate. In a given substance, the Elemental composition varies in proportion. The characteristic Elemental composition of any substance is the material bedrock upon which all other phenomena such as attributes, taste, and actions operate. Each Element contains a subtle half known as its "subtle essence" or *Tanmatra*. This

constitutes a significant nutritional component that feeds the individual on an energetic level.

4. *Rasa*. This Sanskrit term has several meanings; some of which are *taste, plasma, essence,* and *sap*. In terms of nutrition and medicinal substances, *rasa* refers to taste, specifically to one or more of the six primary tastes: sweet, salty, sour, bitter, pungent, and astringent. The concept of taste, in fact, has a corollary meaning; that is, the subjective taste experience evoked within the individual by the ingestion of a food or herb. Dietary and medicinal materials, themselves, however, are considered to have some intrinsic taste qualities, in part, determined by their Elemental composition. Taste or *rasa* in the operational Ayurvedic sense is virtually identified with the nexus between the taste nature of ingested materials and the subjective taste experience that they evoke.

THE NATURE OF TASTE OR *RASA* ACCORDING TO AYURVEDA

Ayurveda places the subjective and objective experience of taste in a premier position. The taste experience, in large measure, is the ongoing, daily, and repetitive contact that the individual makes with the outside world. Satisfaction, pleasure, and survival result. Western medicine has delineated an extensive neurophysiologic mapping of the mechanisms underlying taste and has included the interdependent mechanisms of the sense of smell, the olfactory system, in describing these sensory functions. While a thorough review of this complicated area is beyond the scope of the present work, a brief outline of some basic principles will be given for the sake of perspective and clarity.

The olfactory function, the sense of smell, is considered relatively more important and overriding in the Western view of gustatory experience. Aromas of ingested substances are produced by their volatile components, and picked up by the sense of smell that is experienced as the "flavor" of food. An almost infinite number of distinct flavors are differentiated in the process of ingesting a substance and these are mainly the result of the substance's aromas stimulating the olfactory cranial nerves.

The sense of smell is mediated by the chemosensory system that includes the nasal olfactory neuroepithelium containing olfactory sensory receptors that, in turn, travel through the first cranial nerve, the olfactory nerve. To a smaller extent, the fifth cranial nerve, the trigeminal, is also involved. The smell experience determines the flavor and the palatability of foods.

The gustatory function, the sense of taste, is considered to have important significance but its functions play a relatively secondary role in overall taste perception since Western medicine views olfactory sensation as more overriding in its interplay with the sense of taste. Gustatory coding is believed to consist of gross and of finer discrimination. There are five major groupings of taste buds with taste receptor cells. Four of these are anatomically located on the tongue; the fifth is more diffuse and has sites on the palate, epiglottis, larynx, and esophagus. The sense of taste is mediated chiefly by the seventh cranial nerve, the facial nerve, which has its distribution on the anterior two thirds of the tongue. The ninth cranial nerve, the glossopharyngeal, and the tenth, the vagus, also play a part. These nerves terminate in the part of the brainstem called the nucleus tractus solitarius and produce, according to the Western view, the experience of the two leading tastes, sweet and salty. The other two tastes that are recognized, sour and bitter, result from the combined olfactory and gustatory interplay.

Ayurveda regards the *rasa* (taste) of a substance as the culmination of its integrated blend of *Maha gunas, gunas,* and Elements. In Ayurvedic nutrition, the essence of food is contained in the innate qualities that are experienced as its taste. The meaning of the essence of food is understood as having a dual nature. The apparent material nature of food is considered to contain its gross food essence. This is composed of some combination of the five great gross Elements (*Pancha Mahabhutanis*), which is gustatorily perceived as food's taste or *rasa*. The ingestion of this aspect of food primarily nourishes the physical body.

The other aspect of food's nature is understood to be its subtle food essence. This is composed of the subtle halves of the great gross Elements, the *Tanmatras*. These subtle essences, not directly perceived by taste, are taken in along with the gross food essences. They are also taken in psychologically through each of the five senses (hearing, touch, vision, taste, and smell). These *Tanmatras* are ingested by *Manas* (mind) and contribute to mental nutrition as well as to overall bodily nutrition, especially to that of the *doshas*.

In Ayurveda, therefore, proper nutrition rests solely on the adequate intake of the five great Elements (*Pancha Mahabhutanis*) and their five subtle, energetic essences (*Pancha Tanmatras*). The gross or combustible portions that can be reduced to ash are important but of second order. The reference point in Ayurvedic nutrition is the experience of taste. Nutrition, therefore, is based on a complex delineation of the taste properties of foods. The almost infinite permutations and combinations of differing quantities and qualities of the Elements produce a spectrum of degrees of specific tastes, and these, in turn, combine to produce distinctive subjectively perceived flavors.

Ayurveda considers that it is the *rasa*, the taste of a food or herb when put on the tongue, that exerts an immediate and localized effect. The launching of this process occurs before digestion proper begins. Since the Ayurvedic term *rasa* signifies both taste as well as the plasma of the body, the intimate association between the two pervades a discussion of each and their interdependent functioning. In Ayurveda, the mechanisms of taste begin to operate first through the medium of water (saliva, *Bodhaka Kapha*), then circulate through channels to reach the brain and mind in order to initiate the complicated process of digestion. Taste is the key point of contact and entry of the unhomologous external world into the internal world. The aim of optimal digestion is to facilitate *Agni's* adequate transformation of unhomologous Elements into homologous Elements that are capable of being assimilated and then providing nutrition to support the *dhatus* (bodily tissues).

Ayurveda recognizes six basic and mutually exclusive tastes. Every ingested substance has a predominance of one or more of these tastes. While every substance contains a portion of each of the five Elements, yet only a few predominate just as only a few essential tastes predominate in any one substance. It may seem quite simplistic, if not reductionistic, to use such a seemingly narrow taste range as the foundation for a broad nutritional concept. The Ayurvedic literature recognizes this, and in a conspicuous fashion, distinctly acknowledges the immense complexity involved in the taste phenomena as well as in the taxonomy and mechanisms of *Dravyaguna Shastra*. The descriptions presented here, therefore, represent a basic introductory approach to a very complicated pharmacognosy and pharmacological body of knowledge, which applies to all ingested substances including foods, herbs, and medicines.

Foods and medicines are primarily classified according to their taste composition. The six tastes are Sweet (*Madhura*), Sour (*Amla*), Salty (*Lavana*), Pungent (*Katu*), Bitter (*Tikta*), and Astringent (*Kashaya*). Each taste has an Element, *Maha guna*, and *gurvadi guna* (10 pairs of opposite qualities) makeup. The Elements in the substance are the chief source of nutrition to the tissues of the body. They restore the body's used-up Elements that are dissipated into energy through the metabolic processes. *Rasa* (taste) is the instrument used to ascertain the Elemental composition of a food or herb. *Rasa*, therefore, is understood to be the taste perception of how the Elements combine in a given food or substance.

The *gurvadi gunas* of a substance contribute to balancing the *doshas* of the body especially when these *doshas* are vitiated or aggravated. The influence of these *gurvadi gunas* is so powerful that their action supersedes or overrides the general effects of the overall taste action of a substance. The *guna* attributes, in fact, have significantly greater efficacy and potency on both the physiological and the pharmacological level. The *Maha guna* effect of a substance affects the individual's quality of consciousness. Sattvic substances refine and enhance consciousness, rajasic substances tend to agitate, and tamasic substances tend to constrict. None of these trends acts unilaterally but generally in concert with only one *Maha guna* predominating.

TASTE AND ITS EFFECT ON THE *DOSHAS*

In Ayurveda, one of the primary methods of affecting doshic balance is through the medium of taste. The taste profile of a substance directly affects the *doshas* (*Vata, Pitta,* and *Kapha*) by contributing either to their increase or their decrease. The Elemental dominance of a particular taste is the chief mechanism that causes the rise or fall of a *dosha*.

Each *dosha* has a predominance of two Elements, one of which may be considered primary and the other secondary. *Vata* (propulsion) has Air as its primary Element and Ether as its secondary. *Pitta* (transformation) has Fire as its primary Element and Water as its secondary. *Kapha* (consolidation) is generally considered to have Water as its primary Element and Earth as its secondary.

Vata in the body is increased by foods that have any of the following tastes: bitter, astringent, or pungent. This is due to the predominance of the Air Element in these three tastes. The secondary Elements in these tastes are Ether in bitter taste, Earth in astringent taste, and Fire in pungent taste.

Pitta is increased by foods that have any of the following tastes: sour, pungent, and salty. Each of these tastes has Fire as its primary Element. The secondary Elements for these tastes are Earth for sour, Air for pungent, and Water for salty.

Kapha has substantial amounts of Water as well as the Earth Element. The three tastes that increase *Kapha* with their associated Elements, respectively, are sweet with Earth and Water, salty with Water and Fire, and sour with Earth and Fire.

The tastes that decrease the levels of the *doshas* in the body are the following. Salty, sour, and sweet tastes decrease *Vata*. Bitter, astringent, and sweet tastes decrease *Pitta*. Pungent, bitter, and astringent tastes decrease *Kapha*.

Taste, therefore, contributes to the modulation and functioning of each *dosha*; taste, in effect, has a therapeutic action. Proper and healthful diet and nutrition can only be achieved by the correct matching of one's individual *prakruti* (constitution, body type) needs with the corresponding foods and herbs. These needs include a range of components such as optimal doshic levels, Elements, *gurvadi gunas*, and *Maha gunas*. The essential idea for optimal health is the ongoing maintenance of equilibrium proper to the optimal functioning of the individual's *prakruti*. Daily attention to this is emphasized since daily needs regularly change. This is, in part, due to the natural utilization and dissipation of the aforementioned components for growth, maturation, and development. In addition, a therapeutic need for restoration results from the processes of depletion (i.e., the Elements) or vitiation (i.e., the *doshas*).

An adequate nutritional level of the range of the five Elements is the single most significant and necessary factor needed to maintain overall equilibrium. These five Elements are the building blocks of the *doshas*, *dhatus* (tissues), and *malas* (wastes). Foods provide ongoing nutrition. Herbs act as healing drugs and medications. Proper nutrition and diet customized to one's *prakruti* and doshic needs keep the *doshas* balanced and optimally functioning. This, in turn, promotes healthy tissues, organs, and psychological well-being. Diet, therefore, is directly related to the quality of health and to the disease process. The Ayurvedic concept of nutrition strongly emphasizes these considerations. The nutritional perspective of Western medicine that deals with foods and their protein, carbohydrate, fat, and vitamin components is recognized as important but is not a major focus in the Ayurvedic view.

THE CONCEPT OF *VIRYA*: POTENCY OR ENERGY

All ingested substances have three basic components: *rasa* (taste), *virya* (potency, energy), and *vipaka* (postdigestive effect). As has been described, the phenomenon of taste is a leading descriptor in Ayurvedic nutritional classification. All substances have the additional characteristic of therapeutic potency, and although this is contained in dietary foods, it is most important when considering therapeutic herbs. The taste aspect is more dominated by the influence of its Elemental composition. The *gurvadi guna* qualities accompanying a taste have a range of potential effects, some of which never manifest in the body.

The *virya* aspect, on the other hand, relates to the energy of a substance and to its capacity to produce a significant and substantial effect. The concept of *virya* may be likened to the dual pharmacological concepts of drug efficacy and drug potency. *Virya* is that aspect of a nutritional substance that exerts its primary effect during digestion proper. *Virya*, the dimension reflecting a substance's energetic temperature, is subsumed within the 10 pairs of opposite attributes or *gurvadi gunas* but retains a special position in nutrition and herbology. The therapeutic potency of many herbs, for instance, relates to their *virya* status.

Although the concept of *virya* includes a range of diverse characteristics, the leading attributes identified with it are on a spectrum with designations ranging from hot to cold. The hot end denotes increased potency to activate; and the cold end denotes increased potency to diminish. This reflects the specific action of *virya* on the *Agni,* the transformative energy of the body. A direct effect on the *Pitta dosha* is closely tied into this. This relates to a positive enhancement of the entire digestive process and is an extremely active attribute of any drug. For example, in terms of a hot *virya,* the salty taste is warm, the sour taste is warmer, and the pungent taste is hottest. In terms of a cold *virya,* the sweet taste is cool, the astringent taste is cooler, and the bitter taste is coldest. The bitter taste most powerfully lowers *Pitta dosha* and *Kapha dosha*. The sweet taste most powerfully increases *Kapha dosha* and decreases *Vata dosha*. Lastly, many factors contribute to a *virya* of a substance. These include its growing location, season of growth, harvesting time and technique, handling, age, and processing.

THE CONCEPT OF *VIPAKA*: THE FINAL METABOLIC AND TASTE EFFECT IN TISSUES AFTER PRIMARY DIGESTION

The concept of *Vipaka* (postdigestive effect) in the digestion process as understood in Ayurveda has the sense of digestive cooking and occurs after the primary macrodigestive processes are completed in the gastrointestinal tract. *Vipaka* represents the delayed systemic whole body effect as the end result of digestion. This metabolic conceptualization, part of an entire spectrum of the metabolic–digestive process, is unique to Ayurveda. The *vipaka* effect of a food occurs after all the digestive processes have occurred when the properly prepared nutrients are ready to be assimilated into cells and become part of the tissue substance. *Vipaka* may be understood as the final assimilative process of microdigestion that represents the culmination of the entire digestive process and yields a bottom line cellular effect within the tissues and the organism as a whole. *Vipaka* represents the dynamic action that uses the essence of foods and herbs in a nutritive manner to support and maintain the body. The *vipaka* of a substance is also more powerful in exerting a therapeutic effect on the tissues than is that substance's primary *rasa* or taste.

In summary, as Charaka (c. 700 B.C.) has explained in his medical treatises, *vipaka* is understood to mean that foods with either sweet or salty tastes remain sweet at the culmination of all digestion. This has a cooling effect, significantly contributes to the nutritive buildup of all seven bodily tissues, and aids in healthy elimination. Many tonic substances have this sweet *vipaka*. Foods with a predominantly sour taste produce a sour postdigestive effect that is somewhat heating, contribute to the buildup of all bodily tissues except the reproductive, and produce a small eliminative enhancement. Foods with tastes that include bitter, pungent, and astringent aspects have a pungent postdigestive effect that is heating and does not contribute to the buildup of bodily tissues or to enhanced eliminative processes. Substances whose *vipaka* is pungent are beneficial in that they act as digestive stimulants and help to reduce *Ama*.

THE CONCEPT OF *PRABHAVA*: THE IDIOSYNCRATIC PHARMACOLOGICAL EFFECT BEYOND *RASA, VIRYA*, AND *VIPAKA*

Although Ayurvedic nutrition and herbology are covered in the concepts of *rasa* (taste), *virya* (potency), and *vipaka* (postdigestive effect), the effects of certain foods and herbs transcend comprehension using these categories. When such a substance with a recognizable set of tastes, energies, and postdigestive characteristics does not behave accordingly, it is said to contain a unique *prabhava*. This special action is usually very pointed in its targeted effect and aimed at a specific tissue, organ, or disease. The *prabhava* quality of a substance frequently is related to a unique energy, potency, and hot / cold quality although this is not invariably uniform.

THE SIX BASIC TASTES: THEIR COMPONENTS, EXPRESSION IN FOODS, AND ACTIONS IN THE BODY

Madura: The Sweet Taste

The subjective sense of the sweet taste includes characteristics of being pleasant, mild, full, and flowing. Sweet is composed of Earth and Water Elements, and its main attributes include cool, heavy, and unctuous (a soft, flowing, liquidy feel just short of being oily). *Unctuous* is the English rendition of a traditional Ayurvedic term that has no direct English equivalent. An approximate meaning would suggest the term *moist*. The temperature appellation *cool* refers to *virya*, the immediate energetic effect of taste on digestion. Substances with a sweet taste increase *Kapha* and decrease both *Vata* and *Pitta*. These substances, therefore, have an anabolic and nourishing overall effect on the body, and are associated with satiation of hunger and thirst. This tissue-building effect is termed *brimhana* and is, perhaps, the most essential nutritional component of a healthy diet. Most foods, i.e., carbohydrates, proteins, and fats, have this *madura rasa* as their primary taste. Herbs with a sweet taste and sweet *vipaka* are considered tonic and restorative. In Ayurveda, there are significant correspondences between specific tastes and body organs and emotional states. The sweet taste is associated with the pancreas, the stomach, and the lungs. In addition, there is a correspondence with feelings of satisfaction, well-being, love, and attachment. In excess, dullness, inertia, greed, and greedy desire may be produced. The food groups that primarily contain a predominance of the sweet taste are carbohydrates, sugars, fats, and proteins. This includes dairy products, grains, fats, oils, nuts, seeds, meat, and fruits.

Amla: The Sour Taste

The sour taste produces a feeling of some stinging and puckering in the mouth, and tends to increase salivation. There is an aperient or appetizing, refreshing, and cleansing effect produced. The sour taste is composed of the Earth and Fire Elements with attributes that include slightly heavy, hot, and unctuous or moist. Sour increases *Kapha* and *Pitta* and decreases *Vata*. Foods with an acid content tend to be sour and supply minerals to the body. Some examples of the sour taste found in foods include acid, citrus fruits, acid and nightshade group of vegetables (such as tomatoes, potatoes, eggplant, peppers), spinach, alcoholic beverages such as wine, yogurt, vinegar, pickles, and fermented items. The sour taste strengthens *Pitta* and enhances digestion. The sour *vipaka* also promotes good elimination of wastes in urine and feces. The pacification of *Vata* tends to promote a reduction in spasm and tremor, and may be related to the high mineral content of many sour foods. The sour taste is associated with the small intestine, stomach, and liver. The emotional states associated with the sour taste are described as a feeling of being refreshed and of increased alertness and attention. In excess, envy, jealousy, and irritability are said to be stimulated.

Lavana: The Salty Taste

The salty taste is composed of the Fire and the Water Elements, and has attributes of being heavy, hot, moist, and sharp. Salt also contains a significant portion of the Earth Element. The hygroscopic nature of salt causes it to attract water and facilitate solubility. The salty taste tends to stimulate, soften, and loosen. Digestion and movement are enhanced and elimination is increased. An overall cleansing action is produced. The salty taste is associated with the kidney. The significance of salt holds a special place in all concepts of nutrition. At times under conditions where *prakruti, vikruti,* and the season require, salt's Water Element has a nutritional or therapeutic effect that is cooling and hydrating. Conversely, when conditions require, the Fire Element may exert its predominant effect and heat the body thus increasing *Pitta dosha*. Both these aspects of salt have medicinal and therapeutic implications. It should be added that, although the current Ayurvedic literature does not emphasize the Earth Element in salt, this important and real property has significant therapeutic implications since it may act to decrease *Vata* and increase *Kapha* and so produce a downward or sinking action within the bodily tissues. In proper amounts, the salty taste is considered to have a grounding emotional effect. In excess, it can aggravate *Pitta* and blood, cause premature aging, and cause laxity of the bodily tissues. Psychologically, excesses enhance tendencies toward avarice, greed, and hedonistic pursuits. Foods with a salty taste supply a variety of minerals to the body and include the range of natural salts from the earth and the sea, as well as foods like the variety of seaweed.

Katu: The Pungent Taste

The pungent taste is composed of the Air and Fire Elements and has the characteristic attributes of being hot, dry, light, and oily. The pungent taste is often referred to by the terms *spicy* and *aromatic*. When ingested, pungent substances produce a tingling sensation on the tongue, increase the flow of saliva and other fluids both in the gastrointestinal and in the respiratory tract, and may cause some lacrimation. The pungent taste decreases *Kapha* and increases *Vata* and *Pitta*.

Pungent substances are carminative (reducing flatulence), expectorant (liquefying bronchial secretions), anticoagulant, antiseptic, and enhance digestion by increasing *Pitta* and enhancing *Agni*. Their strongly transformative actions tend to increase catabolism and the reduction of bodily substances (*langhana*). They strongly increase *Pitta* and consequently tend to be very drying. Included in this large group are the spices, aromatic herbs, and some essential oils. The pungent taste is associated with the liver. The emotional aspects produced by and associated with the pungent taste are those related to stimulation and increased awareness. In excess, irritation, anger, and aggression may be provoked.

Tikta: The Bitter Taste

The bitter taste is composed of the Air and Ether Elements. Its basic attributes are light, cold, dry, subtle, and penetrating. Bitter taste reduces *Kapha* and *Pitta* and increases *Vata*. Bitters tend to diminish the flow of saliva and dry the mouth. The chemical vehicles of bitter are the alkaloids and the glycosides. The effects of the bitter taste are pronounced in the body. They include a drying, reducing (*langhana*), catabolic, and purifying effect. The bitter taste is linked with the gall bladder. This taste component strongly stimulates digestion through an enhancement of *Vata*, which has a cleansing action on the digestive process. The bitter taste is strongly detoxifying. The bitter taste is associated with a strong trend toward mental clarity, the opening of consciousness, and a sense of sobriety. In excess, it may produce a sense of coldness felt both physically and emotionally and experienced as grief, sorrow, or depression. The bitter taste is a component of some plant and vegetable substances including some herbs. For example, vegetables that are considered predominantly bitter are dandelion, chicory, endive, and artichoke; most beers are primarily bitter in taste. Some herbs with significant bitter taste aspects include turmeric, fenugreek, and aloe vera. Bitter herbs are noted for their potent *prabhava* effect.

Kashaya: The Astringent Taste

The astringent taste is composed of the Air and the Earth Elements. Its chief attributes are slightly heavy, cool, and dry. The astringent taste produces a sense of stiffening, contracting, and puckering in the mouth and throat, dryness, and reduced saliva flow. The chemical vehicle for astringency is usually found in the tannins. This taste is relatively uncommon and usually consumed in very small quantities. Western medicine, at this time, only differentiates four taste groups: sweet, salty, sour, and bitter; the astringent taste in not considered a distinct taste class. Ayurveda describes the actions of the astringent taste to include those of drying excess secretions, some anti-inflammatory effects, a general healing tendency, and acting to provide some needed minerals. This taste is linked to the kidney. Psychologically, it has been associated with asceticism, and a general reduction of emotionality, fear, and fright. In large excess, astringent foods may cause increased bodily dryness, constipation, possible impotence, and decreased physiological functions. Some common foods and other edible substances that have astringent qualities are cabbages, potatoes, teas, lettuce, sprouts, raw vegetables, some grasses, pomegranates, cranberries, quince, some apples, and unripe bananas.

PRACTICAL NUTRITION: GENERAL DIETARY GUIDELINES

Practical nutrition comprises guidelines (*upayoga samstha*) for the proper preparation and consumption of foods as well as the proper choice of foods based on one's *prakruti*, age, the season, and current needs. The following delineates some fundamental guidelines for an optimal and healthy diet.

1. A balanced diet includes all six tastes to be ingested each day.
2. Dietary choices should be compatible with one's individual *prakruti*.
3. One's diet should generally include foods with qualities that are opposite to one's predominant *dosha* or *doshas*.
4. All foods should be of high quality and should be wholesome (*satyma*).
5. Foods should be fresh; freshly prepared for each meal; and should be cooked and eaten warm or hot. Occasional salads, of course, are eaten raw. The cooking process tends to maximize digestibility and to minimize adverse effects.
6. The largest meal of the day should be eaten around noontime.
7. No food should be eaten until the previous meal has been adequately digested.
8. The quantity and types of foods consumed should match the state of one's digestive fire, the *Agni*.
9. The quantity of food consumed at a meal should be about three-quarters of the stomach's capacity.
10. Incompatible food combinations and improper food mixing should be avoided. The chief examples of this include the following. Milk should not be consumed with any other food except grains. The most undesirable combinations are with bananas, fish, or sour fruits. Eggs should never be eaten with cheese or with potatoes. Melon should always be eaten

alone. Yogurt as well as eggs should also be eaten by themselves. Honey should never be cooked. One should never eat honey and ghee in equal proportion. One should never eat a mix of hot with cold foods together.

11. One should generally avoid eating foods that are excessively heavy and cold or excessively dry.
12. Very cold beverages and iced water are not recommended.
13. One's eating demeanor and setting should be pleasant, congenial, and quiet. One should not eat when emotionally upset, or rushed. There should be minimal talking and maximal focus and concentration on the food and the eating process. One should try to appreciate the eating experience using all five senses. After eating, one should walk for about 20 minutes. One should avoid heavy *Kapha*-like foods such as yogurt, ice cream, and sesame products after sunset. No food should be eaten within 2 hours of going to sleep.
14. Large quantities of yogurt, ice cream, cheese, and meat are not recommended. If consumed, they require the addition of spices to act as "antidotes" to prevent excessive adverse reactions. Some examples of these include the following. Yogurt should be consumed with small amounts of ginger or cumin. Ice cream should be eaten with small amounts of cardamom or cloves. Black pepper or cayenne pepper should accompany cheese. If meat is eaten, some added cayenne pepper and some turmeric will make it more digestible. If alcohol is consumed, cardamom or cumin will counter some of its adverse effects.

Special attention needs to be given to the concept of *satyma* (wholesomeness) concerning foods and herbs. *Satyma,* which embodies a high degree of *Sattva* (essential goodness), refers to the degree of optimal quality and purity that a substance, activity, or process contains. Dietary choices need to be carefully considered since only substances that are *satyma* are beneficial to consume. Foods, spices, and herbs need to be fresh, unadulterated, and not or only very minimally processed. The concepts of "organic," "natural," "free from pesticides and herbicides," "hormone free," and "not genetically engineered" are representative of trends toward *satyma* substances and their production.

AYURVEDIC FOOD GROUPS

Ayurveda recognizes about a dozen different food groups. This differentiation is based on empirical experience and is not necessarily restricted to the carbohydrate, protein, and fat model of modern organic chemistry. The following constitute the Ayurvedic food groups.

1. Cereals and grains (*sukadhanya*)
2. Legumes, beans, and lentils (*samidhanya*)
3. Meat (*mamsa*)
4. Vegetables (*saka,* and *harita varga* for raw)
5. Fruit (*phala*)
6. Nuts
7. Milk and dairy (*gorasa*)
8. Water (*ambu*)
9. Wine and spirits (*madya*)
10. Sugars (*iksuvikara*)
11. Spices, minerals, fats, oils, and condiments (*aharayogin*)
12. Cooked food preparations (*kritanna varga*). This category is made up of various preparations that include soups, fruit juices, and cooked milk products.

AYURVEDIC ASPECTS OF COMMON FOOD GROUPS

Food, in general, supplies basic nutrition to the tissues and to the whole body. As a whole, food is considered to have a primarily sweet taste, a neutral energy, and a sweet postdigestive effect. A commonly accepted modern classification of food groups is the following: fruits, vegetables, grains, beans, nuts, dairy products, meat, sugars, oils, and spices or condiments. While it is beyond the scope of the present work to address all aspects of foods in general and in particular in terms of their nutritional and medicinal qualities, the following brief outline will present a basic overview. Practical cookbooks and food guides using Ayurvedic principles are relatively few in number but available (Douillard, 2000; Morningstar & Desai, 1990).

Most fruits are considered to have a sweet taste, a cool energy, and a sweet postdigestive effect. *Vata* and *Pitta dosha* are slightly decreased, and *Kapha* is increased. This produces a balanced condition if fruit is taken in moderation. In excess, the digestive fire is diminished and *Kapha* may increase to produce excess fluid and, possibly, *Ama*. Fruit is considered to be highly sattvic and pure. Sweet fruits are highly recommended for those with *Vata* or *Pitta* predominance. Fruit in moderation is acceptable for *Kapha* persons. Apples may be the best choice for *Kapha* predominance.

Vegetables are more of a heterogeneous group of foods than fruit. Their taste may range from sweet (root vegetables, for example) to astringent (leafy greens, cruciferous, beans, for example) to pungent (onions, chilies) to bitter (dandelion, chicory, for example), to salty (seaweed), and to sour (some nightshade vegetables). Their energy tends to be neutral, and their postdigestive effect is usually sweet.

Grains are considered to be sweet in taste, neutral in energy, and sweet in postdigestive effect. Basmati rice is considered a balanced grain and beneficial to all *dosha* types. Wheat is heavier and so tends to be more *Kapha* increasing. Barley is a useful grain, especially suitable for *Pitta* and *Kapha* constitutions. Beans are highly *Vata* producing and so are not recommended except to those with strong *Kapha* body types. Split yellow mung beans or lentils are unusual because they are tridoshic (beneficial to all *doshas*), and so are recommended for all. Nuts and seeds are considered sweet in taste, warm in energy, and sweet in postdigestive effect. They are sattvic in nature and are especially recommended for those with *Vata* predominances.

Dairy products are considered to be sweet in taste, cool in energy, and sweet in postdigestive effect. In general, all dairy products tend to be sattvic in nature and very nutritive. Before the modern era, milk was not homogenized, pasteurized, or produced from cows treated with hormone and antibiotic drugs. Animal feed was more organically produced in that synthetic herbicides and pesticides were unavailable. In order to eradicate the transmission of milk-born diseases, pasteurization at high temperatures became a public health necessity. Pasteurization may be necessary nowadays to provide disease-free dairy products on a wide scale. Ayurveda believes that dairy products, currently produced on farms that do not use more natural, organic methods and use homogenization, are safe but substantially less beneficial to health since they contribute heavily to the production of *Ama*. Recommendations are for limited milk use, in general, especially in adulthood. When milk is used, it is suggested that it be warmed to a gentle boil with a pinch of ginger or of turmeric in order to reduce its *Ama* provoking qualities. Charaka has compared the nature of *pure* milk to that of *ojas*, the essence of life, and considered it a major *rasayana* (rejuvenative tonic). Milk is best taken alone, or with some grains (cereals), or with ghee. Milk should never be consumed with fruits, especially bananas. Ghee, which is clarified butter, is one of the most sattvic foods, and is recommended almost unreservedly when used in moderation and in a context of monitoring of blood triglyceride and cholesterol levels and any other obviating metabolic or cardiac concerns.

Meat, chicken, and fish are considered to have a sweet taste, a warm energy, and a sweet postdigestive effect. The ancient Vedics used meat. Ayurveda uses meat and meat products judiciously. Systems of Yoga tend to encourage vegetarian practices since meat is considered rajasic (agitating) and highly tamasic (dulling) in nature as well as contrary to the principle of *ahimsa* or nonviolence. Since meat is a highly nutrient packed food, it will increase *Kapha* if used excessively. It will also increase *Pitta*. Meat decreases *Vata* and may be a part of *Vata*-predominant diets when necessary. Depending on an individual's overall lifestyle and personal preferences, the inclusion of some meat in the diet may be beneficial in order to balance *Vata* excess and to restore a sense of overall grounding. Meat in the form of soups and stews that are cooked with vegetables, oils, and spices into a homogeneous blend are considered best. Since meat (like nuts) is a highly concentrated food that resists easy digestion throughout the gastrointestinal tract, large quantities at any meal are not recommended. Viewing the use of meat more as a condiment may be a good choice. The nature of eggs is a special case of a concentrated food derived from the animal world. Eggs have strong nutritive and reputedly aphrodisiac properties; they may decrease *Vata* and increase *Kapha* as well as stimulate *Rajas*. The consumption of eggs, therefore, is considered acceptable but needs to be judicious and not excessive.

Oils and fats are considered to be sweet in taste, warm in energy, and sweet in postdigestive effect. The best oils and fats for consumption according to *dosha* are the following: *Vata*: all oils, especially sesame and ghee; *Pitta*: olive, sunflower, ghee; *Kapha*: a minimum of all oils; sunflower, mustard, flaxseed, and ghee in moderation are acceptable; a small amount of olive oil may be beneficial. Ayurveda advises that every individual consider judiciously incorporating an appropriate amount of oil and ghee in the daily diet. Substantial elimination of all dietary fats is thought to be unwholesome. All dietary vegetable oils, including ghee, are best consumed uncooked, that is, added in the raw state to foods; light cooking is acceptable. Since heating to high temperatures diminishes the nutritional quality of oils and ghee, they should be consumed in their natural and uncooked state or in as minimally cooked a condition as possible. Animal fats in meat and chicken soups and stews need to be cooked.

Sweeteners are usually recommended for different doshic types. Those with *Vata* predominance may use all types of sweeteners in moderation. *Pitta* constitutions do well with the use of maple syrup since it is cooling. *Kapha* body types may use honey since it is warming and has diuretic properties.

The choice of condiments and food spices depends on constitutional type. *Vata* types may use all spices that are moderate in intensity. Examples of this include ginger, cinnamon, cardamom, cumin, and fennel to name just a few. Salt and vinegar in moderation are also acceptable. *Pitta* body types require only mild spices such as coriander, cumin, cinnamon, cardamom, fennel, and turmeric, to name just a few. Salt and vinegar are not recommended. Those with a *Kapha* constitutional predominance may take all spices in large quantity. Hot and intensely pungent spices reduce excess *Kapha*. Salt and vinegar are not recommended. Coffee and regular teas have some bitter qualities and may be used by all *dosha* types in small amounts without harmful effects. Alcoholic beverages are not forbidden. Excessive use, however, evokes rajasic turbulence and usually increases *Pitta dosha* to an inordinate degree. Some medicinal herbal and wine preparations taken in moderation are beneficial.

DIETARY CHOICES ACCORDING TO *PRAKRUTI*

One's innate constitutional type reflects the predominence of one or more *doshas* and the characteristic qualities that they impart to the structure and physiology of the body. Digestive capacity or *Agni* is one of the major functions of *prakruti.* Dietary food choices, therefore, should be closely aligned with *dosha* predominance. Traditionally, a range of choices has been found to best suit each *prakruti.* While these suggestions have been proven over time, they are not rigidly mandated. They act as guidelines that need to be adapted to the nuances and variations of each individual body type.

Vata-Predominant *Prakruti*

Vata dominant *prakruti* constitutions require dietary regimens that are opposite to the chief attributes that characterize *Vata.* The attributes of *Vata* include cold, dry, light, rough, subtle, clear, mobile and agitating. A nutritional regimen that is opposite to *Vata's* attributes is desirable. Diets should be regular, grounding, and moderately substantial, warm, and moist. Temperature of foods should not be too hot or too cold. Raw foods should be kept at a minimum, especially apples. It is also best to avoid beans, lentils, raw vegetables, cabbages, broccoli, brussel sprouts, lettuce, mushrooms, and dry foods such as popcorn, potato chips, and pretzels. Freshly prepared soups, stews, warm beverages, and moist, moderately oily foods and food combinations are best. The tastes that are best to emphasize in the diet are sweet, sour, and salty.

Foods that balance *Vata* include sweet moist fruits, lemons, mangoes, some cooked vegetables, grains such as basmati rice, oats, and wheat, mung beans, all nuts and seeds, and all oils and fats. All dairy products and all sweeteners, except honey, are good. All spices that are moderate in intensity are recommended, as is a moderate amount of salt and of vinegar. Animal products such as meat, fish, and eggs are good in moderation. Nuts and seeds, however, should be restricted in cases of diverticular disease of the colon.

Pitta Predominant *Prakruti*

Pitta predominant *prakruti* constitutions require nutritional regimens that are opposite to the inherent qualities of *Pitta*. *Pitta* has hot, dry, light, penetrating, and oily qualities. The digestive capacity of *Pitta* types is usually very good, but overheating and overacidity may be a problem. Dietary choices should avoid hot and pungent foods. The following foods should be kept to a minimum: sour and citrus fruits, bananas, nightshade vegetables (tomatoes, potatoes, peppers, eggplant), onions, garlic, hot spices, salt, vinegar, nuts, honey, meat, and lentils; fried foods, peanut butter, and alcohol should be avoided. Foods should be eaten warm or cool.

Pitta constitutions do well on fresh, sweet fruits, most vegetables especially artichoke, celery, asparagus, dandelion, chicory, and escarole, basmati rice, barley, some beans such as mung and chickpeas, oils such as olive and sunflower, ghee, most dairy products, all sweeteners except honey, mild spices such as coriander, cumin, fennel, turmeric, mint, and a small amount of cardamom, and mild light fish and meats (chicken). Raw vegetables and salads are recommended in moderation. Foods that are cooling, light, and calming are best. Sweet, bitter, and astringent tastes should be emphasized in the diet.

Kapha Predominant *Prakruti*

Kapha predominant *prakruti* constitutions are strong, grounded, and robust by nature. The optimal *Kapha* diet should be opposite to the chief qualities of *Kapha;* these are cold, heavy, oily, soft, and dense. Because of the heavy nature of *Kapha,* diets should be light and stimulating. In general, the following foods tend to be heavy and should be minimized: dairy products, meat, wheat, oats, nuts, fats, oils, as well as sweets, salt, and vinegar.

The consumption of heavy, starchy vegetables like sweet potatoes, the nightshade family of vegetables (tomatoes, potatoes, eggplant), and okra should be minimized in general. All cold or iced foods should be avoided.

The best diet for this constitutional type is light, warm, dry, and stimulating. The best fruits are apples, cranberries, and pears; some lemon and some dried fruits are good. Most vegetables, e.g., celery, garlic, onions, cabbage, and green leafy ones, other than the heavier ones such as potatoes, are excellent choices and a *Kapha* dietary mainstay. Grains such as barley, buckwheat, and rye are good. All beans including lentils are recommended. Very small amounts of oils and fats are recommended. Ghee, sunflower, mustard, and flaxseed oils are good choices. The best sweetener is honey. Small amounts of meat as well as eggs are acceptable. *Kapha* types do very well with large amounts of all spices particularly the hotter ones like black pepper, ginger, and red pepper. Pungent, bitter, and astringent tastes should predominate in the diet.

GENERAL DIETARY CHOICES ACCORDING TO THE SEASONS

Although one's diet should be shaped to fit one's basic *prakruti,* seasonal variations play an exceptionally important part in affecting individual *doshas* and the interplay of the *doshas* in the constitution. Each season has its characteristic attributes and qualities, and one's dietary choices should tend to be opposite to the characteristics of the current season. This is an important dietary guideline and, in general, partially overrides or should take greater precedence, to a judicious degree, over dietary choices than choices based on one's constitution alone. An optimal diet tailors one's individual *prakruti* needs with the features of the environment at any given moment.

Ayurveda has divided the year into two broad seasonal periods: (1) *Adana Kala,* a period of relative weakness; and (2) *Visarga Kala,* a period of relative strength for all biological life. In India where there are six seasons, *Adana Kala* occurs roughly from mid-January through mid-July. It is a time of relative dryness and exerts a dehydrating quality to nature and to man. During this period, all biological organisms are relatively weakened, less energetic, have less available strength, and diminished digestive power (*Agni*). This generally hot, dry period is broadly associated with a predominance of solar forces and is called *Agneya*. In the United States where there are four seasons, the window for this period begins at the vernal equinox, around March 21, when the number of hours of day equals that of night; its decline occurs near the end of September well after the summer solstice, around June 22. *Adana Kala,* thus, occurs from spring through summer.

Visarga Kala follows this and goes from the end of September through the end of March. It is a period of increased moisture, less heat, growing strength for both man and other biological organisms, and stronger *Agni*. During this period, for instance, vegetables become richer and more nutrient packed. This span of time has been called *Saumya,* the cooling, moist time of the year dominated by lunar forces. In the United States, it begins at the autumnal equinox, about September 22, and begins to decline at the winter solstice, about December 22, when the sun is farthest from the equator. It ends at the vernal equinox in late March. *Visarga Kala,* thus, occurs from autumn through winter.

Dietary Choices in the Fall

Fall is a *Vata*-dominant season characterized by cool, dry, windy weather that tends to be irregular and changeable. The autumnal equinox, occurring around September 22, is an especially significant junctional transition and is considered an important stressor for man in the Ayurvedic system. The irregular weather changes between hot and humid and then cool and damp are confusing to one's doshic balance and can become severely aggravating and disruptive. All constitutional types, therefore, should tend to employ diets that are cooked, warm, moist, grounding and slightly heavier during this fall season. Foods that are pacifying to *Vata* should be emphasized. Spices that are exceptionally good at this time of year include cardamom, cinnamon, fresh ginger, basil, fennel, rosemary, and asafetida. Asafetida is an uncommon spice in the West but is a common Indian spice. It is very strong in aroma and is used in small amounts.

Dietary Choices in the Winter and Early Spring

Winter is a *Kapha* dominant season characterized by cold, dark, heavy, and damp conditions. There is a pointedly still, constricted, frozen, almost inert quality that pervades these months. All constitutional types benefit from diets that are warm to hot, substantial, and stimulating. Cold weather strengthens the digestive processes, and the *Agni* is enhanced and able to handle heavier foods. Foods that are consistent with balancing *Kapha* should be emphasized. Spices that are best include black pepper, red pepper or cayenne, dry ginger, and sage, to name just a few.

Early spring is the season in which the cold, dense qualities of *Kapha* are beginning to be assuaged by the burgeoning heat of the approaching *Pitta* summer season. Accumulated body *Kapha,* at this time, naturally tends to soften and liquefy. The looming warmth of this season requires foods that are cooler, lighter, less oily, and less sweet and sour in taste. Bitter vegetables such as dandelion, chicory, and artichoke are of great benefit.

Dietary Choices in the Summer

Summer is the time of *Pitta* predominence. Heat and dryness prevail. The digestive powers represented by the condition of *Agni* are diminished at this time. Foods, therefore, should have characteristic lightness, coolness, and calming rather than stimulating qualities. Cooling fruits and some dairy products are best if one is able to digestively handle dairy products. This is the time of year when aloe vera is most beneficial taken both internally and applied externally. Beneficial cooling spices include coriander, some cumin, turmeric, and peppermint.

Dietary Choices at Times of Heavy Rain

Whenever heavy rains occur (spring, late summer, and early fall in the United States; July and August in India), their coolness tends to chill and aggravate both *Vata* and *Kapha*. The dampness, humidity, and possible acidity present in the rain, as well as intermittent heat, tends to aggravate *Pitta*. The heavy rains that usually occur around the autumnal equinox (September 22) are especially distressing because this juncture between summer and autumn exerts the most direct and stressful impact on the individual as a whole. This is related to the weakened condition that normally results from the previous hotter and drier period of the year, and the usual *Ama* buildup from inside the body. At these times of tridosha irritation, the use of honey is ideal. Warm teas to which honey is added are beneficial to reduce dampness and add warmth. Fresh ginger root used in teas and in foods is cleansing and pacifying. Grains such as barley and rice, along with freshly prepared light to medium vegetable soups, are recommended.

DOSHA COMPATIBLE DIETARY CHOICES

Vata Pacifying Diet

General: Warm foods and beverages that tend to be moist and moderately oily; sweet, salty, and sour tastes should predominate.

Fruits: Sweet fruits, apricots, avocado, bananas, berries, cherries, coconut, dates, fresh figs, grapefruit, grapes, lemons, mangoes, sweet melons, oranges, papaya, peaches, pineapples, plums.

Vegetables: Cooked vegetables, asparagus, beets, carrots, cucumber, garlic, green beans, okra, onions, parsley, sweet potatoes, radishes, watercress, zucchini, salads with oil.

Grains: Basmati rice, cooked oats, wheat.

Legumes: No legumes except mung beans, warm tofu, black and red lentils.

Meats: Chicken, turkey, and seafood.
Nuts and seeds: All nuts and seeds.
Dairy: All dairy products in moderation.
Oils: All oils especially sesame.
Sweeteners: All sweeteners except white sugar.
Condiments and spices: Cinnamon, cardamom, fennel, cumin, basil, fresh and some dry ginger, cloves, small amounts of black pepper, salt, and mustard seeds are preferred.
Avoid or reduce the following: light, dry, and cold foods; foods with pungent, bitter, and astringent tastes; barley, corn, millet, rye, buckwheat; dried fruits; raw vegetables, cabbages, broccoli, celery, eggplant, mushrooms, peas, white potatoes, tomatoes; apples, pears, cranberries, watermelon; and all beans.

Pitta Pacifying Diet

General: Warm foods that have a predominantly sweet, bitter, or astringent taste.
Fruits: Sweet fruits; apples, avocado, coconut, figs, grapes, mangoes, pears, pineapples, plums, pomegranate, prunes, and raisins.
Vegetables: Asparagus, broccoli, brussel sprouts, cabbage, chicory, cucumber, cauliflower, celery, cilantro leaves, dandelion, escarole, green beans, leafy greens, mushrooms, okra, peas, green peppers, potatoes, sprouts, small amounts of yucca root, and zucchini.
Grains: Barley, cooked oats, Basmati rice, wheat.
Legumes: All legumes and beans except lentils.
Nuts and seeds: No nuts except coconut; no seeds except sunflower and pumpkin.
Meat: Chicken, turkey.
Dairy: Ghee, cottage cheese, milk.
Oils: Olive, sunflower.
Sweeteners: All sweeteners except honey and molasses.
Condiments and Spices: Coriander, cinnamon, cardamom, fennel seeds, turmeric, peppermint, small amounts of cumin, black pepper, and fresh ginger.

Avoid or reduce highly spiced foods, hot spices; foods with predominantly pungent, sour, and salty tastes; yogurt, sour cream, cheese, buttermilk; honey and molasses; sesame, almond, and corn oils; corn, millet, rye, brown rice; lentils; sour fruits; hot peppers, radishes, tomatoes, eggplant, garlic, onions, spinach, beets; nuts; beef, seafood, eggs; salt; vinegar, and alcohol. Peanut butter is exceptionally *Pitta* provoking.

Kapha Pacifying Diet

General: Light foods and diet that is dry and warm with tastes that are predominantly pungent, bitter, and astringent.

Fruits: Apples are best; apricots, berries, cherries, cranberries, dry figs, mangoes, peaches, pears, persimmons, pomegranates, prunes, and raisins.

Vegetables: Most vegetables are very desirable, especially asparagus, beets, broccoli, brussel sprouts, cabbage, cauliflower, celery, eggplant, garlic, leafy greens, lettuce, mushrooms, okra, onions, parsley, peas, peppers, radishes, spinach, sprouts, and watercress.

Grains: Barley is best; Basmati rice, corn, millet, dry oats, buckwheat, and rye.

Legumes: All legumes and beans except cold tofu.

Nuts and Seeds: No nuts; no seeds except some sunflower and pumpkin.

Meat: Chicken, turkey.

Dairy: No dairy except ghee, goatmilk, and skim milk.

Oils: No oils except sunflower, flaxseed, and small amounts of virgin olive oil.

Sweeteners: No sweeteners except honey.

Condiments and Spices: All spices except salt; dry and some fresh ginger is very beneficial.

Avoid or reduce overeating; avoid foods that are cold and oily, and those with predominantly sweet, sour, and salty tastes; avoid all dairy products and oils other than very small amounts; avoid all nuts and pork; avoid large amounts of beef and seafood.

CHAPTER 9

LIFESTYLE AND BEHAVIORAL REGIMENS, YOGA, AND MEDITATION

AYURVEDIC REGIMENS FOR OPTIMAL HEALTH

Health maintenance is essential for promoting balance and integration throughout the bodily, mental, emotional, and spiritual dimensions of each individual. This presumes maintaining a rigorous reality sense, which constitutes the ability to differentiate in a skillful fashion both the grosser and finer distinctions within nature, to rank their relative positions in the scheme of reality, and to reasonably discern their differing levels of meaning. This discriminative understanding then guides one in selecting and implementing suitable choices within the fabric of everyday living. Ayurveda addresses these needs in its guidelines for food and nutrition (*anna*), lifestyle and behavioral practices (*vihara*), and herbal supplementation (*aushadha*). The Sanskrit word *swastha* means healthy, and the state of optimal health is called *swasthavritta.* This is understood to constitute a "harmonious abiding in one's own nature" and means living in harmony with one's constitution during the changing course of the life cycle as well as that of the seasons. A fundamental sense of satisfaction both psychologically and felt in the body results from increasingly balanced and optimal functioning. The concept of a healthy lifestyle includes particular consideration to three aspects of one's conduct and behavior: (1) *dinacharya,* the daily regimen; (2) *ritucharya,* the seasonal regimen; and (3) *sadvritta,* one's ethical outlook and behavior.

Dinacharya or daily regimens are closely allied to personal hygiene routines. They include optimal times to awake (before sunrise), care of the mouth with special attention to the teeth and tongue, and care of the eyes, nose, ears, and skin. Care of the tongue is especially important and involves routine morning mild scraping with a special tongue utensil that produces both a cleansing effect and a stimulating action. Morning routines include attention to cleansing procedures as well as regular bowel habits, breathing exercises, stretching and Yoga exercise routines, some massage, and bathing.

Ritucharya or seasonal routines include dietary choices and activity recommendations proper to the season. In general, the best time to engage in active exercise is the *Visarga* period in fall and winter. One's strength is optimal at this time. In addition, one's diet should be relatively greater in quantity since all foods are believed to be imbued with greater energetic and nutritional components. The *Adana* period in spring and summer is a time for less exercise and less food intake. This period is considered to be one of diminished overall energy and strength and should be used for greater rest and activities that require less physical exertion.

Sadvritta or ethical regimens include recommendations that examine and address one's values and behavior, especially interpersonal and social aspects. Emphasis on this reflects the importance that Ayurveda gives to areas of one's life extending beyond those pertaining only to the single individual and to the care of the material body. The Ayurvedic literature stresses that these guidelines are not merely considered to be moral dictums nor believed to be solely culturally based. They are understood as universally applicable principles of proper conduct for all people in all circumstances. Ayurveda, by its internal nature, neither discriminates against, rejects, nor summarily excludes differing worldviews either Western or Eastern. Ayurveda is inclusive. It does put exceedingly heavy weight on meditative techniques and consciousness enhancing viewpoints that have a proven record of accomplishment and efficacy. The ancient sages laid unreserved emphasis on this. While the conceptual framework and styles surrounding these do have a distinctly

Eastern flavor, Ayurvedic health regimens, nonetheless, are expressly applicable to all religious, nonreligious, spiritual, philosophical, and humanistic orientations.

Sattvic (pure, balanced, good) qualities in thought, feeling, and action are directions considered valuable to strive toward, embrace, and attempt to achieve. These include self-discipline, proper management of the five sensory faculties, impulse control, regulation of desire, avoidance of harm to self and others, honesty, truthfulness, and working to achieve health in body, mind, and consciousness. All endeavors, therefore, that aim at enhancing refined consciousness, harmony, balance, intelligence, compassion, and mental equanimity are considered to be valuable, meritorious, and in the service of producing excellence.

These proposed healthy lifestyle regimens must arise from an individual sense of personal responsibility for work on the self. Membership in groups or organized bodies that help to facilitate this self-work is always important, although self-work on an individual basis must continue to remain primary. Parents and all caregivers, however, are in vital positions of influence and nurturing. Direction and guidance, especially by modeling, example, and quality, mutually interactive dialogue provide indispensable and organic sustenance for the welfare of the next generation. Child-rearing techniques, accordingly, may find Ayurveda to be a valuable resource. Ayurvedic lifestyle regimens are a well-suited accompaniment to all child care practices.

In due course, a new person, man or woman, one with enlightened wisdom, can be generated thereby. Individuals of this higher spiritual caliber then contribute to the establishment, in a true sense, of a new nation of integral human beings whose real wealth is firmly and rightly established on enduring spiritual insights. Power, influence, and authority then manifest not in relation to others but as the empowerment of the self. Life wisdom thus engendered is predicated on a deep sense of gratitude with heartfelt compassion and is not constricted by historical or theoretical legalisms and narrow dogma. This enrichment, brought about by the deepening of consciousness, can act to raise, in a significant way, the quality of life for all people in every walk of life.

LIFESTYLE REGIMENS BASED ON *DOSHA* PREDOMINANCE

Lifestyle regimens generally address what are considered to be the "three pillars of life": (1) food; (2) sleep; and (3) the management of sexual activity. These represent fundamental and biologically based needs. In addition, we may add guidelines that address occupation, exercise, and aspects of the psychological life of man, i.e., mental health. All recommendations derive from an understanding of *prakruti,* one's constitutional body type, as it operates within a particular environmental context. Guidelines for each of the three primary doshic types are outlined to serve as broad directions to be further customized and appropriately combined in order to suit mixed constitutional types. Since there are, in fact, as many different *prakruti* types as there are people in the world, these recommendations are to be considered as rough blueprints that require ongoing individualized adaptation to changing conditions: stage of the life cycle, season, particular stressors at a given time, etc.

Vata Predominance

The *Vata dosha* (principle of propulsion), considered the strongest *dosha* (bioenergetic principle regulating the body), is also the most sensitive and may easily become disturbed or vitiated. This is true for all *Vata*-dominant *prakrutis,* and for the *Vata* component within all individuals. To maintain balance, *Vata*-dominant individuals require regular meals preferably with the main meal taken around noontime. Smaller regular feedings may be required. This is acceptable since *Vata* innately tends toward variability, which may be addressed therapeutically by habits aimed at regulating the tendency toward irregular, inconsistent behaviors. Foods should be taken warm, moist, moderately oily, and consist of moderately heavy items. Stews or cooked mixtures of a variety of different food items prepared together are beneficial and more easily digested. Fasting should be avoided.

Sleep should strive for regularity. One should awake by sunrise and go to sleep relatively early. Sleeping or naps during the daytime are permitted when necessary. *Vata* becomes aggravated when an individual stays up very late into the night. This is an Ayurvedic fact of exceeding importance. It affects the *Vata* component in everyone and results in a multitude of physical and mental difficulties, which are potentially preventable.

Exercise should be regular and moderate. As is true for all doshic predominances, one should only exercise to half of one's capacity. In addition, when one begins to perspire, exercise should be stopped. Those with *Vata* dominance tend to be driven, hyperkinetic, and prone toward frenetic, maniclike activities. Exercises such as aerobics, running, jumping, and jogging are highly aggravating to *Vata* and are not recommended. Mild, regular activities such as walking, stretching, golf, horseback riding, and sailing are preferable. Tai chi is especially soothing for *Vata*. Yoga exercises will be described later.

To maintain mental health and prevent the natural tendencies toward anxiety, fear, mood swings, mania, and feelings of insecurity, *Vata* types should strive for regular, balanced hobbies, study, and meditation. In addition, the *Vata* component naturally present to some extent in each individual also may be benefited by implementing these trends at times during which inordinate stress exacerbates *Vata dosha*. *Vata*-dominant persons tend to generate original and creative ideas although they require pacing and discipline to remain focused and follow tasks to completion. These people do well in professions that are compatible with this trend. Regular oil massage reduces excess *Vata* in both body and mind, and is highly recommended as a routine practice. The best climate is one that is both hot and humid.

Since specific stresses and activities tend to aggravate *Vata* in very serious ways, the following is a partial list of some main culprits. These include exposure to wind and cold, excess talking, traveling, especially on airplanes, excess exposure to highly stimulating sensory inputs such as television, radio, loud music, cinema, and computers. *Vata* is specifically aggravated by loud and harsh sounds. Regarding sexual activity, it is believed that *Vata* persons require less frequency and degree of intensity than do those of other *dosha* predominance. While the central importance and nuances of human sexuality are an intimate part of life, a detailed survey here is beyond the scope of the present work. It, nonetheless, must be said that this area, innately prone to excesses, is often perceived and dealt with in too casual a manner. Improper management seriously impairs aspects of the *Vata dosha* in all persons regardless of specific constitutional dominance. That disturbance in *Vata,* in turn, causes further turbulent cascades of derangement in *Pitta* and *Kapha.* Judicious attention to this heavily counted area is an important consideration for the wholesome conduct of any lifestyle.

Pitta Predominance

Pitta dosha (principle of transmutation) is associated with the strength of transformation and the penetrating intensity of intelligence. Preferences should be for foods that are cool, calming, and minimally stimulating. *Pitta* predominant constitutions do well when eating salads and a moderate amount of raw vegetables. Alcohol and very hot spices should be avoided. The largest meal should ideally be taken around noontime when *Pitta* is naturally strongest and digestive capacity is optimal.

Sleep is usually sound and regular. A moderate requirement of about 6 hours is usual. If *Pitta* becomes aggravated, sleep may become disturbed with typical awakening at around 1 to 2 A.M.

Exercise preferences usually tend toward competitive sports. This should be avoided since it will aggravate *Pitta.* Sports that are more team oriented or performed alone are preferred. Recommended exercises and sports include swimming, canoeing, sailing, hiking, archery, and skiing; hobbies such as gardening are soothing and beneficial. Tai chi and Yoga are conducive to a balanced activity regimen.

Pitta is the *dosha* of heat, and all things associated with excess exposure to heat are not recommended. Outdoor exposure to the sun, sunbathing, steam baths, and hot climates, in general, should be avoided.

In order to maintain psychological health and reduce irritability, anger, hostility, unduly critical attitudes, inordinate competitivess, and controlling tendencies, *Pitta prakrutis* should try to avoid heat engendering situations (foods, spices, competition, etc.). The *Pitta* predominant person tends toward deep, penetrating intellect and sustained attention toward task completion.

Careers and occupations that require this degree of mental organization, fastidiousness, and precision are *Pitta dosha* compatible, i.e., engineers, detail managers, physicians, attorneys, professors, etc. The best climates in which to live are those that are both cool and temperate.

Kapha Predominance

Kapha dosha prakruti, in balance, is strong, stable, grounded, and steady. Food choices should tend to be light, warm, dry, and stimulating. All cold, frozen, and iced items should be avoided. The main meal should be around noontime, and all food intake should cease by early evening.

Those with *Kapha* predominance require the least amount of daily sleep. Six hours may be sufficient for the adult. Infancy, childhood, and a large part of adolescence constitute the developmental period of *Kapha* dominance. Infants and children naturally require substantially more sleep, and adolescents require no more than eight hours. The adolescent predilection for staying up late into the night and then sleeping into the late morning hours is particularly deleterious and should be carefully monitored and avoided. Parental guidance is advised, if not critically important, in safeguarding the welfare of children and adolescents whose healthy upbringing is predicated on such responsible and vigilant parenting. Awakening by or shortly after the time of sunrise is recommended since it may insure or, at least, create conditions for optimal functioning. This admonition may be the *single most important safeguard* that responsible parents might implement in caring for the young, especially adolescents.

Sleeping during the daytime hours is considered very unhealthy, especially for those of a *Kapha* constitution, since it strongly increases *Kapha dosha.* Staying awake relatively later into the night but going to sleep before or by midnight is acceptable. Since sleep has an intimate connection with the quality and quantity of *Kapha dosha,* those with this constitutional type are especially prone to oversleeping. The negative consequences of this are numerous and result in pervasive lethargy, indolence, and passivity both physically and psychologically. Staying awake late into the night, therefore, is exceedingly deleterious since it not only disturbs *Kapha,* but the added disturbance in *Vata,* i.e., restlessness, impulsivity, and evoking a penchant for thrill seeking activities, compounds the magnitude of the vitiation. When anyone, for that matter, stays awake late into the night, a vicious cycle is set up that predisposes to oversleep in the morning. Sleeping later into the morning hours tends to increase *Kapha* to abnormal amounts and this has a ripple effect that tends to disrupt both *Vata* and *Pitta. Prana Vata* has an intimate connection with clarity of consciousness, fundamental balance, and sound health. Disturbances of *Vata,* therefore, are most important to avoid or minimize.

Kapha dominance is the only *dosha* type that benefits from very intense, rigorous exercise. Strong aerobic exercises, weight lifting, running, jogging, bicycling, as well as all strenuous physical activity is beneficial and recommended. In addition, moderate exposure to the sun and judicious sunbathing are acceptable.

In order to prevent excess *Kapha* from accumulating, *Kapha*-dominant types should avoid exposure to excess cold in foods and environments, too much sleep, procrastination, and inordinate bouts of physical and mental inertia. Psychological health maintenance also will curb *Kapha*'s natural and passive tendency toward lethargy, complacency, greedy and possessive attachments, and depression. Pursuits that are more intrinsically active, such as those requiring stimulating study, travel, and healthy action-oriented pastimes, are most beneficial. This *dosha* dominance performs well in caring, nurturing, counseling, and administrative endeavors. The best climate is one that tends to be hot and arid.

YOGA AND MEDITATION

Yoga and Ayurveda: Their Differing Emphases

The practice of Yoga and meditation may be considered part of the system of Ayurveda insofar as it may complement and enhance Ayurvedic practices. Although they share some similar, yet not identical, origins with some historical parallels, there are important differences between the two. Ayurveda is more ancient and derived from the Vedic foundational texts, particularly the *Rig-Veda* and *Athara-Veda*. Traditional or classical Yoga theory and practice, codified by Patanjali is at least 2,000 years old and thus relatively younger than the Vedas (Condron, 1991; Dasgupta, 1989). Patanjali, author of the *Yoga-Sutra*, the source text of classical Yoga, may have lived in the second century A.D., although Hindu tradition identifies him with the famous grammarian of the same name who lived 400 years earlier. While sharing many similarities, Ayurveda and Yoga contain some significant and qualitatively differing emphases. Whereas the Yoga system has stronger dualistic themes underlying its ideology and practice, Ayurveda tends to be relatively more monistic in that a biopsychospiritual integration is advanced. Yoga systems tend to suggest trends toward ascetic renunciation (*tapas*) of the flesh and of the material world (Condron, 1991; Dumont, 1980; Kaelber, 1989; Olivelle, 1992). Ayurveda, on the other hand, puts more positive emphasis on the physical body and the material aspects of the environment as they contribute to health and well-being. In many ways, Ayurveda can be regarded as having a more "full bodied" rather than "disembodied" espousal of all aspects of life and living. This robust emphasis on the positive value of the body within nature is primary.

Among the goals of Ayurveda, a central theme is the attainment of a healthy and progressively purified body since it is the physical aspect and expression of its mental and consciousness dimensions. When the body is maintained in optimal balance, psychological and spiritual experience is enhanced. A delicate balance between being in the world versus being identified exclusively with the world, i.e., materialism and hedonism, restructures in a positive sense the meaning that attachment (*upadana*) to material reality plays in the Ayurvedic worldview. Although man's spirituality is considered primary and significant, Ayurveda's first attention begins with spirit's material counterpart, the physical body. The Vedic goals of life, personal and social duty (*dharma*), necessary material wealth (*artha*), sexual and material pleasure (*kama*), and enlightenment (*moksha*) are intrinsic to Ayurvedic values. While Ayurveda is the basis for the practice of a healing profession, the application of its principles and values by individuals in a personal way can optimize general health and overall well-being in all aspects of daily living.

Yoga, on the other hand, is a self enhancement system primarily practiced by the individual, mostly in a private manner, as the decisive method for self-development and spiritual advancement through purification of body and mind (Eliade, 1973; Mishra, 1959, 1963; Sarkar, 1993; Vishnudevananda, 1960). Unlike Ayurveda, Yoga disciplines are usually not a primary means for health maintenance and addressing specific medical problems and illnesses. In Yoga systems, more emphasis is given to mental and spiritual hygiene, disciplining the mind and enhancing consciousness, per se. In the initial stages of Yoga studies, i.e., *Hatha* Yoga, a familiar and commonly pursued activity virtually synonymous with Yoga in the West, physical postures (*asanas*), breathing exercises (*pranayama*), and, perhaps, an attempt at meditative practices (*sadhana*) constitute the entire Yoga practice. Advanced Yoga techniques (*samyama*), while incorporating the aforementioned preliminary procedures, lay much greater emphasis on mental training, deepening constraint, and the refinement of consciousness. While Yoga practices allot ample attention to the needs and care of the physical body, the meditative experience, taming of the inherently unstable mind, and rigorous disciplining of the senses, constitute the highest values and become the primary focus of work. The literature of both Ayurveda and Yoga, however, shares common terms and has a similar conceptual and theoretical framework although the emphases, methodologies, and procedures of each differ.

Yoga: Its History in the Ancient Vedas and Later Development by Patanjali

In a manner similar to that of Ayurveda, the historical roots of both Yoga and meditation originated from Vedic sources (Feuerstein, 1998). Precise historical dating relating to the development both of Ayurveda and of Yoga including its meditative practices is ambiguous at best. Yoga emerged later and, therefore, has a relatively more explicit written textual rather than oral foundation. The ancient Vedic origins of Yoga can be traced using later Vedic texts. The Upanishads (c. 600 B.C. to 300 B.C.) appear to contain explicit and clear references. The earliest Upanishad, the *Brhadaranyaka,* may contain the earliest historical reference to meditation in its description of admonitions for the stilling of the mind in order to concentrate its focus inwardly for the purpose of perceiving the true self or spirit (*atman*). Although there are many early references, historians consider the first use of the term *yoga* to have occurred in the *Katha Upanishad.* This early work also relates a classic metaphor that embodies the sense and aim of the yogic pursuit.

In a famous dialogue between a man named Nakiketas and the personification of death, Yama, man is likened to a chariot driven by horses and steered by the individual person. The chariot represents the body, the horses represent the senses, and the charioteer represents the self or spirit. In this analogy, the life of man is seen as a journey powered by potentially wild and unbridled instincts that require discipline and guidance in order to insure a direct path to a destination. The destination is reached by the journey to the core of the self that transcends the ordinary state of merely existing in the world in an unquestioning and nonintrospective manner. The highest value is considered to reside in the deepest understanding of the true nature of the self, and this, in turn, becomes identified with an understanding of the ultimate nature of all existence.

The famous epic literature of India, the *Mahabharata* (c. 400 B.C.–A.D. 300) as well as the *Bhagavad Gita,* contains descriptions of Yoga practices and of schools with differing emphases such as the pursuit of knowledge (*jnana*), of action and service (*karma*), and of love and devotion (*bhakti*). The most famous of the Yoga Upanishads (c. 100 B.C. to A.D. 300), the *Yogatattva,* describes four kinds of Yoga: (1) *mantra yoga,* the repetition of sacred sounds; (2) *laya yoga,* the activation of the *Kundalini* energy that enhances consciousness; (3) *hatha yoga,* the practice of body postures and breath control; and (4) *raja yoga* (the best or royal yoga), which became the comprehensive system *later* elucidated by Patanjali and his school (c. 100 B.C. to A.D. 500). The pre-classical Yoga schools before Patanjali emphasized the goal of individual union and identity with the universal, immanent spiritual ground of existence.

The modern-day system of Yoga practice is essentially derived from Patanjali's *Yoga Sutras* (Condron, 1991; Feuerstein, 1989). These writings codified the classical Yoga system as we know it today and outlined what were considered its eight limbs (*ashtanga*). This series of mental and physical practices were aimed at purifying consciousness by disciplining the naturally wandering mind and training it to become more focused and singular (*ekagrata*). This activity over time would then lead to a union or *yug* between individual consciousness (*atman*) and the universal consciousness (*Purusha, Brahman*). The result of this is the state termed self-realization (*samadhi*). In turn, liberation and enlightenment (*moksha*), in fact, complete transcendence (*kaivalya*), a total separation from the material world, would be achieved. Classical Yoga, therefore, seeks extrication from the material world in contrast to Ayurveda's emphasis on embracing, purifying, and refining the material dimensions of experience.

The eightfold path of union, the *Ashtanga Yoga*, was comprised of the following in ascending order of refinement or purity of consciousness.

1. *Yama,* mental restraint and ethical interpersonal behavior. The five fundamental guidelines included *ahimsa* or nonviolence, *satya* or truthfulness, *asteya* or not stealing, *aparigraha* or nonoverindulgence and detachment from material and worldly things and activities, and *brahmacharya* or regulation of sexual experience.
2. *Niyama,* personal observances, practices, and disciplines. These included cleanliness and purity of body, senses, and heart; serenity and contentment, austerity and ascetic practices (*tapas*), study of sacred texts (*svadhyaya*), and devotional surrender to the highest good (*bhakti* and *prapatti*).
3. *Asana,* physical Yoga postures.
4. *Pranayama,* the intentional and regulated control of breathing in order to normalize it, and thus, in turn, quiet and still the mind.

5. *Pratyahara,* the withdrawal of attention in the sensory faculties from their outward sensory objects.
6. *Dharana,* narrowing the mind by focusing and concentrating.
7. *Dhyana,* the process of meditation.
8. *Samadhi* or *Satya Buddhi,* the ultimate union of the microcosmic self with its origins, macrocosmic consciousness. *Kaivalya,* total extrication from matter, is *samadhi's* superlative achievement.

The system of Yoga in all its variations and differing modalities is a time-honored endeavor to help regulate, enhance, and develop body, mind, and consciousness. It was devised to highlight and address the natural unruliness and untamed quality of the mind, its passions, inclinations, and oftentimes unhealthy life choices. It continues to be a necessary and beneficial path for those to whom it provides the suitable vehicle for serious self-examination and work. Although Ayurveda and Yoga are qualitatively different disciplinary fields, they are compatible and can be mutually enhancing. As was alluded to previously, there are both some obvious and some more subtle differences. In order to further explicate the differences that are significant yet more subtle, some nuances of each will be highlighted. This may help to distinguish each in terms of its respective general perspective, emphases, metaphysical values, and material practices.

Yoga as a discipline stresses a contemplative and meditative mode of experience and action. In its metaphysical worldview, Yoga begins with a strongly dualistic frame of reference. This view sees man as a potentially realized self who needs to overcome his inherently unstable and disorganizing tendencies. The worldly environment, in effect, is viewed as potentially hostile. Aspirants on the Yogic path, therefore, may see themselves as strivers or even warriors struggling to fight and oppose bondage (*bandha*) to the sense objects of the material world. Yoga practices aim at controlling, disciplining, and virtually eradicating the range of desires and power of the bodily instincts that fuel desire and thus perpetuate worldly attachments. Renunciation is given a high value. It is achieved by *tapas,* i.e., rigorous discipline, mortification, asceticism, and *dhuta,* which is the gradual shaking off of all aspects of bondage to the world. The idea of the continual striving for detachment to worldly experience pervades traditional Yoga systems. There is a subtle sense of this constituting an underlying negative world bias or socially negating attitude. The strict self-discipline (*samyama*) that concentration, meditation, and striving for *samadhi* requires connotes a progressively introspective journey. The ultimate achievement is called *kaivalya,* that is, the absolute liberation from connectedness to anything. Purity, in the Yoga sense, is equated with the withdrawal of the spirit from the flesh. The Yoga of Patanjali was profoundly associated with the formalization of ascetic and renunciate cultural movements. This, in part, may be interpreted as having been a "reaction formation" taken to extremes as a result of the innate difficulty of managing oneself with equanimity in a diverse world in which pleasure, wealth, envy, greed, desire, and human frailty was (and is) part of daily living. Classical Yoga systems offered a means of addressing this problem. This classical separatist paradigm, however, had exceptions, notable of which was the Integral Yoga school (Aurobindo, 1976) advanced by Sri Aurobindo (1872–1950).

This characterization of such a subtle propensity in Yoga, it is hoped, is not meant to oversimplify or reduce the profundity and value of the contribution that Yoga has made to man's striving for meaning and self-development. The main thesis of the contrasts between Ayurveda and Yoga, however, does have a firm basis in the substantiated history and texts of the Yoga tradition. Along with the significant contributions to personal development and well-being that Yoga philosophy and procedures have made and continue to provide, one is impressed with an indisputably fervent spiritual and, at times, almost antimaterial or other worldly leaning pervading the classical Yoga corpus. Recognizing this, accordingly, in the context of the immense contributions that Yoga and its practices have made to man's search for meaning and self-development, its judicious integration, in a balanced and complementary fashion, into Ayurvedic health practices can only enhance, if not strengthen, the value of both approaches. The renowned Ayurvedic physician, Charaka, in his foundational medical text *Charaka Samhita,* has extolled the merits of Yoga practices as being conducive to the attainment of *moksha* (enlightenment and freedom).

YOGA PROCEDURES ACCORDING TO *DOSHA* PREDOMINANCE

Yoga procedures include Yoga postures (*asanas*), breathing techniques (*pranayama*), and purification practices (*shuddhi kriyas*). There are specific postures and breathing techniques that are suitable for maintaining the health of the body and contributing toward the balancing of doshic irregularities. Some of the more important of these that are specifically applicable to the three broad classes of *prakruti*, the *Vata, Pitta,* and *Kapha* constitutional types, will be outlined. A full elaboration of the six yogic purification practices is beyond the scope of the present work, but they will be mentioned in brief. They have their parallel in the Ayurvedic *Panchakarma* system of intensive bodily purification, which will constitute a complete discussion later. Since the scope of Yoga practices is broad and includes a vast vocabulary unique to its own point of view and system, only simple English terms will accompany their Sanskrit equivalents in the text. These, along with other terms specific to Yoga theory, will not be included in the glossary but can be found in other texts devoted to Yoga practices (Condron, 1991; Mishra, 1959, 1963; Vishnudevananda, 1960). The *Shuddhi Kriyas* comprise the following six procedures:

1. *Neti,* nasal cleansing
2. *Dhouti,* stomach cleansing
3. *Nauli,* abdominal contractions
4. *Trataka,* cleansing the eyes
5. *Basti,* enema cleansing (not therapy) of the colon
6. *Kapalabhati,* forceful exhalation, abdominal contraction, and inhalation

Vata-Dominant Constitution

The *Vata*-dominant *prakruti* requires procedures that are mild to moderate in intensity and have regular, relaxing, and stabilizing features. Some beneficial Yoga postures include the *sukhasana* (easy pose), the *siddhasana* (perfect pose), and the *padmasana* (lotus pose). These three *asanas* help regulate the *Vata* subdoshas of *Prana* and *Udana*. The *shavasana* (corpse pose) balances all the *Vata* subdoshas, and the *vajrasana* (kneeling pose) helps regulate the *Apana Vata* subdosha. The best breathing technique is the *nadi shodhana pranayama* (alternate nostril breathing). The *nauli* (mild abdominal contractions) help *Samana Vata* subdosha. *Apana Vata* subdosha is responsive to Yogic *basti*.

Pitta-Dominant Constitution

The *Pitta*-dominant *prakruti* requires procedures that are moderate in intensity and tend to be cooling and calming. Some beneficial Yoga postures include the *bhujangasana* (cobra pose), the *sarvangasana* (shoulder stand) that helps regulate *Pachaka Pitta*, the *halasana* (plough pose) that helps *Ranjaka Pitta*, and the *shirsasana* (headstand) that helps *Sadhaka Pitta*. The *shitali kumbhaka* (cooling breath) is a very gentle and beneficial breathing exercise. Another breathing technique, done in great moderation to avoid overly cooling the body, is called *chandrabheda* (lunar *pranayama*) and consists of left nostril breathing techniques. The *Alochaka Pitta* subdosha is benefited by the cleansing techniques of *trataka* and *kapalabhati*.

Kapha-Dominant Constitution

Kapha predominant *prakrutis* require strong, intense, and forceful procedures. The *suryasana* (sun salutation exercise) and series of postures, the *paschimotasana* (sitting with forward stretching posture), and the *yogamudra asana* (symbol of yoga posture) are all helpful for *Kapha dosha*. The best breathing exercise is *suryabheda pranayama* (solar breathing). This is especially useful for regulating the *Avalambaka Kapha* subdosha. Other useful breathing techniques include *ujjayi* (loudly victorious breathing) and *bhastrika* (bellows breathing) technique. *Dhouti* stomach cleansing benefits the *Kledaka Kapha* subdosha. *Neti* (nasal cleansing) helps the *Bodhaka Kapha* subdosha.

THE *TANTRA* OF AYURVEDA: VISION, MISSION, AND METHODS

Ayurveda may be understood as having strong tantric features. *Tantra,* a Sanskrit term, is broadly defined as a system characterized by wefts of technique and a fabric of complexly interwoven mechanisms that incorporate significant use of the life force (*Prana, Kundalini*) to promote integration and achieve degrees of self-actualization. Charaka defines *tantra* as a garland or wreath of interconnected topics that adorn and display the Ayurvedic corpus. This "path that liberates from crudeness" implies a unified strategic base both ideologically and practically. An action modality such as this rather than a contemplative mode characterizes Ayurvedic practice. The precepts of Ayurveda are principles of understanding and rules of conduct. Putting health regimens into action is essential. Ayurvedic wisdom denotes the incorporation of its views and principles into the fabric of everyday living. Not only are the choices of specific activities of daily living more consciously selected, but their very enactment becomes an engagement that is more consciously savored.

Ordinary or conventional experience is viewed as naturally tending to be faulty and continually subjecting the individual to imbalanced states. Since this is seen as a regular and expectable occurrence, it is actively embraced with positive therapeutic enthusiasm. Rather than addressing man's imperfect states with an attitude of opposition, Ayurveda, in this way, becomes deeply involved with and initially accepting of these impure and disordered conditions of suffering and pain. Suffering, in this sense, may be considered to be a normative, natural phenomenon within the dynamic interplay of health maintenance. It may be understood to act as a spur eliciting self-development and an advance in compassion and empathy, which connotes an extended social benefit. Seen in this light, suffering provides an opportunity rather than a misfortunate closure; man's will and his capacity for choice can thus be exercised. In addition, a consideration of the problem of evil, both natural and manmade, from this angle, perhaps, may broaden insight into this vexing and often troubling phenomenon.

The original Vedic prescription for a balanced life stressed adherence to self-discipline through prescribed action within mainstream society. Enacting dharmic responsibilities and obligations maintained the *bandhu* (harmonizing balance) between man and extended nature, the animate and inanimate environment. Man's purpose in life was and is considered to include active participation with great nature, *Prakriti,* in the ongoing dynamic processes of reparation and creation, i.e., healing, restoring balance, and bringing freshness to the self and the world at large. Life, in this sense, was and is considered to be a moral task.

History, personal and social, to be sure, is the arena within which *Prakriti* grows, matures, and develops. God, in this sense, is immanent within, not split apart from, history and the world. If the meaning of *dharma* is understood to encompass aspects of one's inherent destiny, then it is conceivable to entertain the prospect that to discover human nature would be to discover human destiny. The purpose of man's life then would reside in the spirit of his nature, which is a reflection of the wisdom and meaning inherent in greater nature. Uncovering this and aligning the two, microcosm and macrocosm, would contribute to the fulfillment of human destiny. In some sense, this may appear to be tautological; nonetheless, it is an idea worthy of further consideration. An essential aspect of Ayurveda, then and now, continues to reside in the goal of transforming less refined into more refined states of being by active adaptations to ongoing changes such as, for example, chronological age, diurnal cycles, and seasonal shifts. Purity, in the Ayurvedic sense, is the ongoing effort to purify the *dhatus* (tissues) of accumulated impurities in order to make living more comfortable and optimal.

Consistent with the *Rig-Veda*'s predominantly worldly view, Ayurveda's recognition, acceptance, and willing penetration into the material world continue to reflect those axiomatic values. A strong sense of the sacredness of the body and of the physical world, including social agencies, gives Ayurveda a world affirming quality and world embracing tone by its ongoing efforts to transform naturally occurring imbalances into more sattvic (pure, harmonious) and balanced states. The deep oneness underlying all apparently diverse manifestations within experience is emphasized, and the microcosmic and macrocosmic interplay within nature is reverently acknowledged. Ayurvedic care, in general, requires consultation, evaluation, guidance, and coaching from a highly qualified Ayurvedic practitioner or physician so that an appropriate dietary, lifestyle, and consciousness enhancing program may be constructed. Active self-care is thus supported and augmented.

SOTERIOLOGY: A CONTEMPORARY REAPPRAISAL AND CONTRIBUTION

Soteriology, the examination of paths and means to salvation, reconciliation, redemption, and enlightenment, has always been an important concern within the domain of visions of man, both Eastern and Western, that include the spiritual dimension (Anandamurti, 1993, 1994; Eliade, 1978, 1982; Forte, 1990; Gurdjieff, 1963; Lamm, 1986; Mead, 1895, 1913; Osho, 1994, 1995, 1996; Steiner, 1964, 1968; Urbach, 1979; Yogananda, 1946; Zaehner, 1961). If we regard Ayurveda as being embedded within a worldview whose conception admits of the existence and reality of multiple experiential dimensions, particularly those of consciousness and spirit, then a consideration of the soteriological implications within it is important to explore. A theoretical framework outlining some major principles and practice guidelines will be given. All substantial work toward spiritual development and the refinement of consciousness, however, requires dedication and the assistance of a qualified teacher or guide in the context of an appropriate setting over time.

In the broadest sense, Ayurveda's *tantra* encompasses a range of activities that are imbued with powerful reparative aims and ends. The ancient Vedic seers (*rishis*) were keenly aware of man's spiritual origins, recurrent ills, pain, suffering, the problem of evil, and need for an organized system of reparation both ideologically and technically. The Vedas provided dharmic mandates for the regular ordering of life through prescribed observances. Spirituality was thus integrated into daily life, which expressed itself as a practical religion of social immersion in the world of everyday living. Goals, values, and purpose in life were applicable to all in general (*samanya*). Life's meaning was embodied in the acceptance and implementation of the four Vedic aspirations: *dharma* (duty); *artha* (material possessions); *kama* (pleasure in living); and *moksha* (ultimate liberation or salvation). The Vedics, however, recognized that all individuals are born and develop in unique and differing ways; therefore, as individual *karmas* (actions and their consequences) vary, so do individual destinies. Individual choices as well as a number of extraindividual influences were believed to combine in unique ways to create one's particular path in life.

While all of the Vedic goals were considered opportunities for everyone, it was recognized that *moksha*, a choice potentially available to all, may not be, and usually is not, universally chosen as an active pursuit. It required an essential and volitional impetus. This impulse may emerge, perhaps, out of an innate longing to know the truth of one's own being, a state of mind with cosmic connotations and existential ramifications. The nature of *moksha* clearly is complex both conceptually as well as experientially. It is certainly not a negligible sentiment for those who experience its stirrings. It has been loosely regarded as being a state of freedom, particularly from blind bondage to *Prakriti* (the manifest and material world), to the cycle of *samsara* (repetitive rebirth into the phenomenal world of impermanence), and to the driving forces of forgetfulness, desire, and ignorance that perpetuate these attachments. However true this understanding may be, it risks being incomplete without further examination.

The ancient Vedic corpus unfalteringly maintained the truth, reality, relevance, and necessity of man's immersion in society and in the material world. Ayurveda still holds this to be true. Using an epistemological perspective that is also consonant with Buddhist thought, a broad description of the processes of thinking will be given as a backdrop for an interpretive contribution to the meaning of the highest of these ancient values, that of *moksha*.

Within the experiences of everyday life, man, interacting with and a participant in the social order, makes sense of the world initially using the ideational process termed *samvritti-satya* or conventional, relative, everyday thinking. This mentation, although complex in its detailed nuances, may be understood to include sensation, perception, concept formation, logic, memory, and reasoning. This given mode of thinking is that aspect of "mind" associated with the Eastern concept of *maya,* the erroneous or incomplete interpretation of the meaning of reality; nonetheless, it may be considered to be a relatively valid and necessary human faculty vital to successful adaptation. A broader, more profound understanding of *maya,* in fact, recognizes that the world, both inner and outer, is the real manifestation of *Prakriti* (nature), the creative base of reality that dynamically unfolds as the human as well as the extended universe. Material realities, therefore, although incomplete in themselves, are not, in fact, nonexistent, false, or artificial. The Western concept of "idolatry" (false objects of worship) reflects the Eastern idea of *Maya* and *prajna-aparadha. Maya,* then, in this perspective, may be recognized not as a deceiver but as the *Great Teacher,* a stern yet gracious entity offering repeated, diverse, and fresh opportunities as well as challenges in the course of one's life trajectory.

Samvritti-satya, however, is the epistemological process that puts a ceiling on cognition, limits its range, and the scope of its depth thereby truncating knowledge, reason, interpretation, and belief. This is the meaning of the Vedic concept *prajna-aparadha,* the mind's inherent cognitive fault that predisposes to errors in wisdom and to forgetting the essential unity underlying the integration of the entire universe. Yet since *samvritti-satya* constitutes the commonsense cognition that contributes to the maintenance of communal integration and order, it has natural value and is useful. It is the means well suited for achieving an understanding of and adherence to the dictates of *dharma, artha,* and *kama.* In fact, since the natural world, particularly the social order, has "real" value, whatever position or walk of life one finds oneself occupying either psychologically, socially, or even geographically is the precise location where the journey toward *moksha* must begin.

In order to achieve degrees of *moksha,* the present author submits *now,* as the sages had done in the past, that *samvritti-satya* needs to be expanded to include the deeper and broader level of awareness termed *paramartha-satya,* an awareness of the existence of the ultimate truth upon which *samvritti-satya* rests. This ultimate truth, which encompasses a dynamic spectrum of varying degrees of deepening understanding, is arrived at initially using thoughts, concepts, and ordinary mental reasoning processes, but extends beyond these. The technique suggested here entails total immersion into the experience of conventional reality using astute perception and exquisitely developed sensory receptivity. For example, an important first step would be to curtail the activity of talking; speaking should occur only when truly necessary. This consequently would contribute to an enhancement of sensory perception, which would become increasingly receptive and thus play a greater role in cognition. Rather than bypassing and blurring the distinctions that are part of everyday thinking, one would begin to develop a keener awareness of an experiential universe filled with crisp and meaningful qualities and attributes, a virtually infinite array of both grosser and more subtle nuances and meanings.

Since the given, natural state of the undeveloped mind is likened to an agglomeration of wild, unruly, and passion driven impulses, a concept akin to the image of a mob of thugs, developing this more random condition into an experiential field with more detail and order must undergo an evolution that, of necessity, would expand over time. It does begin, however, with self-inquiry and within the very psychological and geographical space that one currently occupies. Ultimately, one's apprehension of oneself within the world could then begin to become realized in a more nonconceptual way. Discursive reasoning would gradually become supplanted over time by a burgeoning intuitive apprehension that is hallmarked by more immediacy and coherence.

Self-inquiry, working on the self, in this mode may uncover the opportunity for a deeper analysis of self that could further delineate one's true nature, the fundamental *prakruti.* One's basic constitution and its vicissitudes over the course of one's lifetime (*karma*), i.e., temperament, habits, defense mechanisms, character, style, preferences, likes, dislikes, etc., would be increasingly more accessible. Leading questions that would emerge are: Am I willing to face hidden, unacceptable aspects of myself? What are these? Can I fully acknowledge and begin to accept these? To the extent that I can do this, what are strategies for change and improvement?

Such direct experiential states, moreover, open one to the proposed idea of a transcendental unity immanent throughout reality. Meditative techniques such as described here can further enhance one's frame of mind. Meditation, therefore, acts to augment any currently held pursuit, worldview, or faith thus introducing more clarity, depth, and strength. In fact, one would be encouraged to remain, at least initially, in one's current life space and to attempt to maximize ongoing engagements in personal, social, and occupational activities of daily living in order to optimize these everyday interactions. Introspective, spiritual, and other contemplative pursuits, as well, could become enriched.

A detailed elaboration of the aforementioned two cognitive–experiential processes is beyond the scope of the present work. *Paramartha-satya*, however, can be understood to be the discernment and insight achieved initially by specific intellectual, emotional, and physical disciplines, which subsequently become restructured by the transcending influence of meditative awareness. This is hallmarked by a state of contemplative receptivity, a silencing of "mind" in Eastern terms, which connotes a condition of experiential immediacy, a sense of being totally present in the here-and-now. This state has been described as one of being in the "eternal now," i.e., timelessness, and, in fact, as being a state of virtual "mindlessness." The latter, it is believed, reflects more refined levels of consciousness and aspects of what in traditional Eastern thought is called "enlightenment," an experiential phenomenon that, in part, denotes the meaning of *moksha*. Mentation, therefore, becomes augmented, purified, and refined by meditative awareness. An innate intelligence (*buddhi*) is uncovered that brings profound wisdom (*prajna*) and compassionate empathy (*karuna*) to the fore. A deeper appreciation of and for the self and a more natural, ethical concern for others emerge. This profound experience of gratitude reflects the process of creative reparation throughout the breadth of one's being.

Moksha, then, becomes experienced as a gradually evolving state characterized by the satisfaction of a range of basic needs that include the epistemophilic instinct for clearer understanding, the achievement of a sense of security and trust in the self and in extended nature, and an approaching feeling of serenity, peace of mind, and contentment. Repeated states of meditative awareness become a surrendering of one's mind in the limitless containment of meditation. Cognitive dissonance recedes. This comes to have a considerably normalizing effect on the natural instability, turbulence, fluctuations, unreliability, and propensity for intellectualization that characterize ordinary mental processes (*vritti*). One becomes more able to engage in the details and practical tasks of everyday living with a keener focus, absorption, enthusiasm, and sense of renewal. One's overall cognitive functioning and its content undergo a transformation. Conventional knowledge becomes enriched by a deeper knowledge, one enlightened by an expanded, spiritualized consciousness. This, in turn, becomes further enhanced as it is imbued with degrees of the ultimate wisdom (*prajna*) that self-realization and self-actualization bring. *Prajna,* the wisdom that *moksha* engenders, has been called "the ultimate medicine."

A deep purification is set in motion that results in the defragmenting of disparate ideas and the organization of more stabilized thought patterns, which contribute to clearer thinking and mental equipoise. The Sanskrit term *anubhava* connotes the transition from an initial state of abstract, theoretical knowledge toward a more direct, authentic, almost intuitive, experiential awareness, i.e., a gradual yet inclusive penetration in meaning from surface to depth. In its entirety, it connotes the development of *prajna* (wisdom). It is to be remembered, however, that these states are, in fact, ongoing dynamic experiential processes. They are relative, relational, and developmentally sensitive. They can be understood to be more attitudinal in nature rather than being final or terminal ends. Psychological development from birth to death undergoes recognizable stages spurred on by physical growth, neurophysiological maturation, and psychological experience. Each stage provides the individual with differing cognitive and emotional faculties. The earlier stages absolutely require the care and guidance of a nurturing figure. This is an ideal time for caregivers to expose children and adolescents to the range of Ayurvedic lifestyle principles, especially those of *sadvritta* (values and ethical behavior). From adult life on, the individual becomes increasingly more self-reliant for basic and extended survival. While the refinement of consciousness can occur to varying degrees at all stages, adult life is usually the time when the impulse for self-examination emerges on a more solid basis. This experiential capacity develops over time and, in part, is related to psychological maturity. Although aspects of this more refined state of mind can be present, to some extent, at any age, it is more commonly achieved later in life, usually after the 40's. The Zen concept of enlightenment and self-realization termed *kensho* aptly connotes this state of developing awareness that gradually deepens over time.

Meditative awareness may begin with isolated periods of meditation and then proceed to become more pervasive and to be experienced as more enduring. It becomes a state of mind incorporated, at first, into a part of one's daily routine and then eventually imbues all parts of every waking moment; meditative awareness becomes the very act of living life to its fullest. It would not be incorrect to understand meditative awareness using the Western concept of prayer in the sense of its being "prayer of the heart," although profound, meditative awareness and expanding states of consciousness, by definition, contain a lightness that is natural, playful, and evocative of a sense of joy. The literature left by great masters of the Buddhist and the Hindu traditions is replete with descriptions of *samadhi* (meditative absorption) and *nirvana* (profound identification with the Absolute) that suggest experiential states that are amusing, cheerful, awe filled, wondrous, and having childlike qualities. The fulfillment of *dharma,* then, becomes an experience characterized by naturalness, spontaneity, and the sense of adventure.

Why some choose to become aware of the possibility of *moksha* and to strive for it remains a mystery. Ordinary man, with his given, mundane, everyday awareness, is described by Eastern and some Western traditions as being passive and machinelike. The nature of "self" in this sense is believed to consist of fragmented, ephemeral aggregates of reflexive thoughts that, for the most part, are evoked randomly and automatically by constantly changing conditions both internal and environmental. The possibility, however, of self-development, in fact, authentic self-creation beyond this mechanical and reflexive ordinary state of mind, is considered achievable. The present work not only continues to advance and endorse this view, but also is an attempt to contemporize its recognition and demonstrate its suitability for modern times.

The proposed shift from being more passive to becoming more active requires radical change, intentionality, and sustained effort. Man's will to change must prevail. The transition to this new state often requires a mental shock to galvanize its organization. This entails an initial recognition of one's utter helplessness in the face of enormous complexity and the infinitely unknowable universe. A willing surrender to this is essential. This attitude may have its roots in the oceanic feeling of infantile oneness that accompanied the developmental fact of primal helplessness. To whatever extent this attitude of surrender is rooted in innate, human phylogenetic memories and the most profound preverbal experiences of infancy as well as earliest childhood is clearly acknowledged. These etiological conjectures, however, neither diminish the importance of this attitude nor make it less radically meaningful. Faith, in this sense, is understood as nascent trust, confidence, and reliance on the intrinsic goodness of the self within nature, and a faithful adherence to the pursuit of self-development. Preeminent focus, nonetheless, must continue to rest on individual accountability and responsibility for personal advancement. Recognizing and pursuing *moksha,* then, amounts to a voluntary covenant with sacred nature understood to be one in essence with self and the extended universe. The dynamics of this voluntary choice constitute a self-election to the path of self-development. This evolves into a veritable self-creation. The distinguishing feature of free choice, then, is axiomatic to the pursuit of *moksha* and enlightened consciousness.

Since the multidimensional roots of such a qualitative change are, in fact, beyond comprehension, one may only begin to launch the process of change by attempting to create conditions within which actual, substantive change, by means of its own inherent powers, will begin to consolidate. If change is viewed as being a dynamic process having an infinite spectrum of activity, then its first stages might aptly be described as a getting ready for change. In this preparatory phase, the obstacles, barriers, and resistances that emerge might best be addressed through a loving engagement. Acknowledging and gently courting apparent impasses, especially under the guidance of a qualified helper, can act, in a gradual manner, to dematerialize these inevitable stumbling blocks. Such therapeutic strategies, needless to say, are complex and require expert handling tailored to an individual's needs at each moment in the process of change.

Pursuing *moksha,* therefore, must include intentional choice along with the emergence of other apparently nonspecific and seemingly random etiological factors. Implicit in this conception is a clear acknowledgment of the influence of the spiritual, the consciousness basis of existence. The phrase *God's will,* in fact, may be related to, if not identical with, this consciousness-based, inherent intelligence within nature. The incommensurability of this, of necessity, leads us to continue to lay exceeding emphasis on whatever part *man's will,* his free will, plays in the mysterious processes underlying the pursuit of *moksha.* The interplay and subtle concordance between these two fractal dimensions, however, must be underscored.

The broad means used to achieve varying degrees of *moksha,* therefore, encompasses an active striving to include wholesomeness (*satyma, kushala*) in all aspects of living, i.e., diet, daily routine, exercise, recreational activity, work, study and learning, meditation, and interpersonal and social relations. Incorporating Ayurvedic principles and practices into one's life enhances all aspects of daily living and raises the qualitative caliber of optimal engagement in the world. These means of striving for ongoing purification, balance, and optimal living may initially require enormous determination and so be experienced as requiring ongoing "superefforts." As a result of this work, however, previously built-up *karma* is deconstructed. This brings about dissolution of the accretions, knots, and layers of concealment (*samskaras*) incurred over time. Corruptions in the experience of the authenticity and purity of the self are detoxified, and both a reparative and creative restructuring is set in motion. The processes of sensation and perception gain more clarity, the repertoire of thinking becomes less rigidly constricted by the characterological defense mechanisms erected by past traumas, and, in effect, mood and affective demeanor become more stable. The unhealthy splitting processes characteristic of *Manas* or mind, including the impoverishing effects of the envy dynamic, diminish, and this softens the proverbial contrasts between dogma versus deed and faith versus reason. The adamantine chains (*samsara*) of past habitual, repetitive and unwholesome modes of experience and behavior (*samskara*) fueled by inordinate desire are loosened.

Not only does this increase in psychological integration make the experience of the ineffable meaning of the self more majestic, but it enhances a less egocentric attitude toward others, one that is more kindly, respectful, and tolerant, if not enthusiastic, in regard to perceived differences. The roots of bias and interpersonal hatred have fear and envy at their base. Self-inquiry and self-development contribute to the progressive refinement of the coarser elements within human nature, the enhancement of consciousness, and the path toward *moksha*. These act as medicines to heal malignant emotional states and as nourishment to vitalize moral consciousness. While concepts such as contrition, repentance, and atonement are more proper to the spiritual traditions of Western religions, their meaning within an Ayurvedic worldview suggests the recognition of imbalanced states emerging by both commission and omission, a personal sense of distress, and the individual resolve to restore harmony.

Over the course of time, previously experienced intentionality in efforts aimed at achieving this newly created disposition toward wholesomeness gradually transforms. An experiential state begins to emerge that is characterized by increasing receptivity, acceptance, and ease. More relaxed, effortless action comes about and a natural spontaneity emerges from this more integrated advance. A biopsychospiritual galvanization is gradually produced that uncovers the engendered awareness of a personal foundation (*atman*) of absolute purity (*Purusha*). This newfound self-realization, then, becomes an integral part of everyday living and ushers in a higher overall quality of life that is experienced more consistently over time. As the natural and limitless breadth of consciousness is felt with increasing conviction, perceived helplessness in all its guises—inordinate arousal, anxiety, fear, and the defensive sense of danger—reconfigures. One becomes grounded in the safety, simplicity, and wonder of experiential witnessing. An inner security is felt as a sovereign presence.

Although words can only meagerly describe the elusive and virtually unfathomable meaning of *moksha,* it can be thought of as the zero point experience termed *Avyakta* (beyond being and non-being), and equally as the positive realization of identity with infinite potentiality or *Brahman* (the Absolute). *Moksha,* then, appears as the felt and sustainable experience that one has always been *Brahman*. The Sanskrit expression *Tat Tvam Asi* (Thou art That), found in one of the oldest Upanishads, the *Chandogya* (c. 500 B.C.), denotes this fundamental Vedic maxim. *Tat* is a very ancient Sanskrit term literally meaning "that" but implying the unknowable principle constituting the foundation of the entire universe, that is, the Absolute.

Moksha, thus, is understood to be the direct, intuitive, and nonconceptual sense of identity with the transcendental Absolute experienced as pure consciousness yet commensurate with an individual's level of biopsychospiritual development. The quality and character of this experiential dynamic may be understood to be a developmentally progressive (not regressive), healthy advance. This mastery is the gain achieved by sublimations that result from conscious and intentional work. Its virtue and value are ensured by the underlying reparative and creative impulses that add to the enrichment of the breadth, depth, and scope of one's consciousness. This insight, it is suggested, is the mutative element within the root meaning of *moksha.* The broad scope of Ayurveda with its engaging presence provides a means to achieve both physical well-being and the liberating, spiritual advancement referred to as *moksha.*

CHAPTER 10

AYURVEDIC THERAPIES, *PANCHAKARMA*, AND MATERIA MEDICA

AYURVEDIC TREATMENT: THE RANGE OF THERAPEUTIC INTERVENTIONS

The range of treatments in Ayurveda is broad and comprehensive. It includes dietary, herbal, lifestyle, behavioral, psychological, meditative, exercise, Yoga, and *Panchakarma* therapeutic interventions (Joshi, 1996; Lele, Ranade, & Qutab, 1997; Ranade, 1993). *Panchakarma* is a group of five specialized techniques used to cleanse and detoxify the body of *Ama* (toxins) and vitiated *doshas* (bioenergetic regulatory substances). The entire spectrum of Ayurvedic therapy, however, aims at restoring the normal balance and functioning of the *doshas*. This entails attention to optimizing the digestive fire or *Agni*. In addition, treatments as well as daily routines for health maintenance attempt to reduce accumulated *Ama* and to prevent its initial buildup. The matrix of treatment rests on proper nutrition and this serves as a base upon which all therapeutic interventions are structured. Restoring balance, therefore, coupled with customized nutritional and lifestyle prescriptions covers the scope of all treatment.

As with the classification of disease and the assessment of diagnosis, the range and nuances of specific therapies can be immense and complex. A brief survey, therefore, with only an orienting discussion will be presented here. A brief but representative discussion of commonly encountered clinical presentations and their treatments from the Western and Ayurvedic perspective will be found in Appendix 3.

BRIMHANA AND *LANGHANA*

The famous Ayurvedic physician, Vagbhata (c. seventh century A.D.), categorized all treatment in two broad categories: (1) *Brimhana* (tonification), and (2) *Langhana* (reduction). *Brimhana* methods tonify, nourish, strengthen, enrich, fortify, and supplement. The term *tonification* is widely used in most contemporary herbal texts to describe the range of these toning, enriching, supplementing, and nutritive interventions. *Brimhana* therapy is also termed *santarpana* (therapy that is indulgent and that gladdens). The primary Elements of Earth and Water constitute the predominating Elements of the substances used since they contribute to an increase in substance, mass, and the *Kapha dosha* (principle of consolidation). The *Brimhana* category has three subdivisions: (1) *Brimhana* (tonification proper); (2) *Snehana* (oleation); and (3) *Stambhana* (astringent therapy).

Therapies that tonify aim at increasing body weight and strength. They are used in conditions that include debilitation, weakness, convalescence, and malnutrition. *Vata* (principle of propulsion) disorders tend to cause weakness and are most responsive to tonifying procedures. *Pitta* (principle of transformation) disorders may sometimes benefit from supplementation, but *Kapha* (principle of consolidation) disorders usually do not require this type of treatment. Tonification or toning therapies are contraindicated in conditions marked by inordinate toxicity, *Ama*, or fever. Diets that tonify are rich and nutritious, and include foods such as milk, ghee, raw sugar, almonds, and rice. Some herbs with marked toning properties include ashwaghanda, shatavari, bala, and amalaki. A lifestyle with little stress, very gentle exercise, and rest is recommended.

Snehana therapy uses oils and fats both internally and externally. Ayurveda stresses the importance of an adequate intake of fat, as, for example, in the form of ghee, olive, and flaxseed oils to maintain proper nutritional balance. When various cleansing and detoxifying procedures are done, large doses of prescribed, medicated oils are taken along with specific external oil massage routines. *Vata* disorders are particularly responsive to oleation. Some *Pitta* disorders require mild oleation. Disorders characterized by significant *Kapha* excess are not treated with oleation since this will intensify *Kapha* and thus exacerbate the *Kapha* condition.

Stambhana or astringent methods are less commonly used in therapy. When used, they act to stop or limit excess discharges from the body such as in bleeding disorders, hemorrhage, or diarrhea.

Langhana or reduction therapies include three subtypes. They are (1) *Langhana* (reduction proper); (2) *Rukshana* (drying); and (3) *Swedana* (sudation). *Langhana* therapies make use of three major Elements: Ether, Air, and Fire. These contribute to processes that reduce, break down, detoxify, and cleanse the body of excess accumulations, toxins, and vitiated *doshas*. Since these reducing procedures are somewhat rigorous, require self-discipline, and may be experienced as difficult, *langhana* treatments have also been referred to as *asantarpana* (therapy that demands abstinence and is discontenting).

Reduction therapy proper (*langhana*) has two major and clinically significant subdivisions first enumerated by Charaka (c. 1000 to 760 B.C.), considered the father and one of the greatest of all Ayurvedic physicians and scholars. They are *Shamana* (palliation, alleviation), and *Shodana* (purification). *Shamana* procedures are commonly used as a part of everyday health maintenance. They are also used in more highly specific ways as individualized treatment interventions and as preparatory procedures before *Panchakarma* (radical detoxification therapy). *Shamana* therapy aims at reducing toxic buildups of *Ama* and vitiated *doshas,* and at supporting the *Agni*. Palliation may be divided into seven methods:

1. *Agni dipana,* stimulating the digestive fire. This is a central and fundamental procedure used therapeutically and for ongoing health maintenance. A number of herbs are used for optimizing the energy of the *Agni*'s optimal transformative power (*dipana*). Herbs that are mild include fennel and calamus; stronger herbs include dry ginger, plumbago, turmeric, and the combination called *Trikatu,* a famous Ayurvedic digestive formula containing black pepper, pippali, and dry ginger.

2. *Ama pachana, Ama* digestion and detoxification. This is another central and fundamental procedure used both therapeutically and for maintenance. There are several herbs used to burn *Ama,* but the main ones are dry ginger, black pepper, and gentian.
3. *Khust,* fasting from food
4. *Trit,* fasting from water or limiting fluid intake
5. Exercise and *Yoga*
6. *Atapa-sevana,* exposure to sun and heat
7. *Maruta-sevana,* exposure to wind and fresh air

Shodana, intensive purification, specifically refers to *Panchakarma* therapy. This is the premier set of techniques that Ayurveda employs to radically eliminate excess vitiated *doshas.* This is usually done under supervision in a therapeutic setting. It is a series of specific treatments with a circumscribed course ranging in time from about 10 days to one month for completion. It will be discussed at length later.

Rukshana (drying) consists of ingesting foods and herbs that may have diuretic properties in addition to the use of dry massage with herbal powders. *Kapha* diseases such as obesity and diabetes are partially responsive to *rukshana* interventions.

Swedana (sudation, fomentation, and sweating) refers to therapies that induce an increase in body heat and cause subsequent sweating. This may involve external applications of dry heat or steam, or the ingestion of herbs such as ginger, cinnamon, and the compound *Trikatu. Vata* conditions marked by cold and dryness are responsive to steam applications. *Kapha* conditions that are cold and damp respond to the ingestion of herbs that have hot and dry qualities.

The two major therapeutic categories, *Brimhana* and *Langhana,* with their six subdivisions as outlined above, have been called *Shad Upakramas* or sixfold treatment. These three pairs of contrasting therapeutic methods cover the entire field of Ayurvedic treatments.

PANCHAKARMA AND AYURVEDIC MATERIA MEDICA

Ayurveda historically has been and currently remains an empirical science. As "life wisdom," it is first and foremost pragmatic in outlook. Its theoretical propositions guide its clinical application. The direct implementation of theory, in a concrete fashion, applied to man living in the world, is the premiere goal-directed action of Ayurveda. As previously outlined, there are a variety of treatment modalities and preventative methods commonly used to maintain health and correct imbalanced states. *Panchakarma*, however, is considered the ultimate treatment, unique to Ayurveda. Unlike *shamana* (palliative therapy) that may be a part of one's daily health maintenance home routine, *Panchakarma* is considered *shodhana* (radical purification therapy) and, in fact, requires the close supervision of a qualified Ayurvedic physician. Many procedures need to be performed in the monitored confines of an Ayurvedic clinic. This therapeutic environment becomes an interpersonal space that is protective, caring, empathic, sensitive, and nurturing. These psychologically sensitive conditions foster efficacious treatment since all aspects of the person are given due and appropriate attention.

CLASSICAL *PANCHAKARMA*

Classical *Panchakarma* treatment consists of three phases: (1) *Purvakarma*, preparatory actions; (2) *Pradhanakarma*, the five principal actions of *Panchakarma* proper; and (3) *Paschatakarma*, also termed *Uttarakarma*, post-*Panchakarma* actions.

Purvakarma

Purvakarma, the first phase of the *Panchakarma* process, is essentially a series of *shamana* (reduction) procedures. These preparatory activities have several objectives. These include reducing and destroying as much *Ama* as possible, increasing the gastric fire (*Agni*), calming and reducing vitiated and excess *doshas*, and then allowing these processed *doshas* to flow back from the compact body tissues (*shakha*) to the more central areas of the body, namely, the gastrointestinal tract and the lungs (*koshtha*). These preliminary procedures thus permit the vitiated *doshas* access to centrally located anatomical areas from which *Panchakarma* proper can eliminate them.

Dietary and Herbal Preparations and Behavioral Recommendations

Purvakarma consists of three parts: (1) dietary and herbal preparation and behavioral recommendations; (2) oleation (*snehana*); and (3) sudation (*swedhana*). Although precise prescriptions can only be given for a particular and individual patient undergoing treatment, a very general outline suggesting customary treatment trends will provide a map showing direction and landmarks. Preliminary procedures usually begin about two weeks before *Panchakarma* proper. The dietary component requires the patient to consume a light diet that avoids heavier foods such as meats, dietary fats, and complex carbohydrates. Light soups of Basmati rice and vegetables are best. A monodiet of *kitchari*, a mixture of Basmati rice, split yellow mung dal (lentils), and mild spices, such as cumin, coriander, turmeric, and fennel seeds, is often suggested. If possible, one should avoid unnecessary drugs, medications, alcohol, and all nonprescribed dairy products. Selected herbs that reduce and destroy toxic *Ama* buildup are consumed. Some representative ones are the following: ginger, black pepper, cumin, chitrak, asafetida, and red pepper. Herbs, such as ginger, fennel, and pippali, which optimize the digestive fire (*Agni*), are also given. This therapeutic dietary and herbal cleansing is essential to target the *Ama* impurities present in cells and tissues in order to neutralize or "burn" as much *Ama* as possible. Any *Ama* residing in the gastrointestinal tract also needs to be detoxified in this way. At this stage, two important preliminary reducing actions are accomplished: (1) attempts to decrease and to destroy as much *Ama* as possible; and (2) optimizing the gastric fire (*Agni*) in order to improve metabolism thus preventing further *Ama* production.

Rest, relaxation, avoidance of exercise and exposure to cold and wind are highly recommended in order to therapeutically curtail any excess actions of *Vata*. One is advised to stay warm, consume warm to hot foods and beverages, and avoid all cold foods and environmental conditions.

Snehana: Oleation

With the above *shamana-purvakarma* procedures in place for at least one week, the next step entails attempts at reducing, calming, and mobilizing the vitiated *doshas* that reside in and are bound pathologically to the tissues. The two primary methods used to accomplish this are oleation (*snehana*) and sudation (*swedhana*). This step is a critical juncture in the attempt to mobilize lodged vitiated *doshas* that are embedded in the tissues. This pathological amalgamation requires this therapeutic series of interventions to disengage the vitiated *doshas*.

The oleation process consists of both the internal (*abyantar*) consumption of oily substances and their external (*bahya*) application. This step has been classically referred to as "turning the wheel of dryness into the wheel of life." The therapeutic ingestion of ghee is used in most cases since it both calms excess *Vata* and increases *Agni*. Other oils such as sesame, flaxseed, sunflower, or mustard, to mention only a few, may be used depending on the specific case to be treated, especially if the clinical condition requires a more heating or drying intervention. Factors such as constitutional type (*prakruti*), the nature of the imbalanced *doshas*, and the season are taken into consideration when making individualized selections concerning the use of specific oils.

Ghee (clarified butter) has been used in Ayurveda for thousands of years. Ghee is butter that is cooked in order to remove both its initial water content (20%), and its milk solids. This renders it relatively stable, lactose free, and able to keep indefinitely without added preservatives or refrigeration. Its use has been considered therapeutic rather than dietary although it has many essential and beneficial nutritional functions. According to Ayurveda, ghee plays many vital roles in the body. Some of its more important functions include (1) stimulating and optimizing the *Agni* (digestive fire, metabolism); (2) reducing all three *doshas*, especially *Pitta* to normal levels; and (3) promoting longevity, intellect, memory, strength, eyesight, and the soundness of the integumentary or skin system. The taste of ghee is considered to be sweet, its energy is cold, and its *vipaka* (postdigestive effect) is sweet.

Ghee is a pure, nonhydrogenated fat about one-third monounsaturated and about two-thirds saturated consisting of about 90% short-chain fatty acids. This profile suggests that it can be beneficial to health since the preponderance of short-chain fatty acids is known to bring about full assimilation and metabolism resulting in energy production. Saturated long-chain fatty acids found in animal fats and red meats, on the other hand, have been shown to be associated with cardiovascular disease, blood clots (thrombosis), and a proneness to carcinomas. Monounsaturated fats, moreover, have been demonstrated to be associated with the prevention of heart disease and cancer. Transfatty acids, found in hydrogenated fats and margarine, have been positively associated with the development of coronary heart disease; ghee contains no transfatty acids. Elevation of the low density lipoprotein (LDL) fraction of blood cholesterol is believed to be one of many (e.g., smoking, hypertension, obesity) major risk factors for atherosclerotic cardiovascular disease. While beneficial fats in the form of essential fatty acids such as fish, flax, and some plant-derived oils are nutritionally necessary, the total saturated fat intake should not exceed between 7 and 10% of all dietary calories.

For safe and salutary dietary and nutritional maintenance, up to one to two teaspoons of ghee per day is suggested; this may be added to food or taken with herbal preparations and preferably should be uncooked. Each teaspoon contains about 45 calories. For therapeutic oleation *on a short-term basis,* about 1 to 5 ounces per day in the morning on an empty stomach is customary; this requires drinking hot water or hot ginger tea during the entire course of the oleation procedure. These suggestions for ghee ingestion are for those who have no specific cholesterol or triglyceride abnormality, no cardiovascular disease, and who have obtained clearance from a qualified medical doctor after appropriate physical examination and laboratory investigations.

External oleation is termed *snehana* when it is used as part of a therapeutic procedure such as *purvakarma.* Some examples of other terms for oil massage that are less medically oriented are *abhyanga* (whole body), *shirodhara* (oil drip to forehead), and *shirobasti* (oil retention on top of head). For external oleation a variety of types of oils is used depending on the specific conditions involved. Some representative oils used are sesame, almond, castor, coconut, and ghee. Small amounts of essential oils having specific therapeutic properties may also be added to the aforementioned for an enhanced *dosha* balancing effect (Miller & Miller, 1995).

Oleation, especially by internal ingestion, serves two principal functions: (1) protection of retainable body tissues; and (2) loosening and separating the vitiated *doshas* from the healthy retainable body tissues. Although some degree of oleation is therapeutically necessary, it is used with caution in those with strong *Kapha*-dominance, obesity, and significantly reduced *Agni*.

Swedhana, Sudation

The last step in the *purvakarma* process is sudation (*swedhana*). This sweating therapy usually involves the application of external heat in the form of steam applied on a daily basis after external oil massage. On occasion, some internally heating herbs, such as ginger, may be given to induce diaphoresis. There are numerous types of sudation techniques devised to achieve heating up of the body and a mild to moderate rise in temperature. Sensitive areas of the body such as the head and the genital areas are protected from excess heat. The two principal objectives of *swedhana* are: (1) to dilate the channels of circulation (*srotas*); and (2) to liquefy the already loosened excess and vitiated *doshas* in the tissues so that they may begin their centripetal flow back into the more central areas of the body. Although some degree of sudation is therapeutically necessary before *Panchakarma*, it is not used or used with great caution in the following situations: *Vata*-dominant constitutions; *Pitta*-dominant constitutions; *Pitta dosha* aggravation and imbalances, especially bleeding disorders, pregnancy, menstruating women, chronic alcoholism, and diabetes.

In summary, *purvakarma's* actions, therefore, include detoxifying the body of *Ama*, increasing the *Agni*, calming vitiated *doshas,* and separating the vitiated *doshas* from healthy bodily tissues. Subsequently, there is a dilatation of the channels that aids in facilitating the vitiated *doshas* in their return from the more peripheral tissues to the central part of the body in order to eventually be eliminated by *Panchakarma.* The means to achieve this includes specialized diet, herbs, oleation, and sudation. During this almost 2–week process, the patient is advised to rest and refrain from exercise. This helps to decrease the activity of *Vata,* and thus add to the overall calming effect of the treatments. A day before *Panchakarma,* the patient is given a more specialized provocative diet called *adhishyandi.* This is specifically geared to increase the targeted vitiated *doshas* to high levels on a temporary basis immediately before the radical *Panchakarma* procedures that will promote their total elimination.

***Panchakarma* Proper**

The second major phase of classical *Panchakarma* is *Panchakarma* proper (five primary therapeutic actions) that constitutes the basis of Ayurveda's core therapeutic interventions. These five actions or procedures include a range of direct and indirect forms and variations of a number of procedures. They are: (1) *vamana* (emesis); (2) *virechana* (purgation); (3) *basti* (enema), two types; (4) *nasya* (intranasal applications of herbs and oils); and (5) *rakta moksha* (blood purification). Charaka (c. 1000–760 B.C.) regarded the first four procedures as fundamental and subdivided *basti* into two types: (1) *niruha basti* (herbal decoction enema) and (2) *anuvasana basti* (oil enema). Thus, he described five procedures with no emphasis on *rakta moksha.* The later work of Sushruta (c. 660 B.C.), the great Ayurvedic physician who specialized in surgery, laid emphasis on the specialized technique of *rakta moksha* along with the other therapeutic *Panchakarma* measures.

Panchakarma is the basis of all purification (*shodhana*) protocols; its aim is an in-depth extirpation of the vitiated *doshas* contained in the channels (*srotas*), the tissues (*dhatus*), and at the cellular level. Before a more in-depth discussion of the five principal *Panchakarma* procedures, some preliminary ideas about Ayurvedic Materia Medica or herbology and indications for *Panchakarma* will be reviewed.

Ayurvedic Materia Medica

The range of *Panchakarma* techniques, like those of *shamana* (therapeutic attenuation of imbalances), involves both physical bodily manipulations and the administration of herbal preparations. Ayurvedic Materia Medica (*Dravyaguna Shastra*) is a blend of pharmacology and pharmacognosy whose origins extend back thousands of years with developments up to the present time.

Since *Panchakarma*, *shamana*, and Ayurvedic Materia Medica are complex, intricate, and finely detailed, not only in theory but also in clinical application, the present text will address only some of the major theoretical principles that underlie them. Aspects of technique and some examples of frequently used Ayurvedic herbs will be mentioned. These represent only highlights and, of necessity, will omit other central and significant procedures, nuances of treatment applications, as well as the extensive and broad range of Ayurvedic herbology that may be found in currently available English texts (Lele, Ranade, & Qutab, 1997).

INDICATIONS FOR *PANCHAKARMA*

Panchakarma, Ayurveda's most radical purification treatment, is given only to those who are relatively strong, healthy, and whose age and constitutions are resilient and able to endure the rigors of such intensive procedures. The range of less intensive, palliative techniques known as *shamana* is a more suitable course of treatment in the following cases: childhood, older age, pregnancy, and severe disease states, i.e., diabetes, hypertension, alcoholism, drug addiction, thyroid imbalances, malignancy, immune deficiency, as well as in postsurgical patients, to mention only some representative examples. Maintaining purity of the tissues is central in Ayurveda, and is accomplished by both *shodhana* and *shamana* therapies.

The three most important indications for *Panchakarma* are (1) health maintenance; (2) treatment of acute disease, and generalized systemic healing; and (3) preparation for rejuvenation therapy (*rasayana chikitsa*). In Ayurveda, health maintenance requires that the normally cumulative amounts of *Ama* be periodically reduced and eliminated from the body using strong eliminative *Panchakarma*. In addition, factors such as chronological age, changing seasons, and normal as well as inordinate life stressors contribute to producing *dosha* vitiation on a regular basis. *Doshas* inevitably undergo unfavorable exacerbation at the junctures of seasons, especially the fall and the spring. At these times, *Panchakarma* is particularly useful. Periodic *Panchakarma* helps cleanse the system of toxic accumulations of a variety of impurities and rids the body of excess *doshas* that contribute to imbalanced states. *Panchakarma* in its health maintenance aspect is considered one of the best available preventative programs to insure optimal well-being. With increasing age, the quantity and quality of vitiated *doshas* and *Ama* in the tissues (*dhatus*) increases; these amalgamated *doshas* lodge in intricate ways. A *Panchakarma* treatment most often removes only a portion of the many layers of embedded impurities. Repeated *Panchakarma* treatments go progressively deeper to remove more obstinate impurities caused by both material imbalances and the *samskaras* (imprinted conditioning over time) that result from past psychological trauma and conflict.

Panchakarma as a disease or *dosha* imbalance treatment is useful in some acute disease states. An acute exacerbation of asthma is one example. Although treating some acute disease states is a classical theoretical indication, it is not customarily done since *Panchakarma* is a powerful and involved technique that requires preparation, professional expertise and application, and a definite period of time. In other words, acute conditions often arise in an unplanned manner; whereas *Panchakarma* is usually an elective and planned procedure. Its therapeutic actions, therefore, may result in healing that is nonspecific but broad in range.

The last major indication for *Panchakarma* is its being the preliminary cleansing procedure that precedes formal *rasayana* or Ayurvedic rejuvenation programs. The elimination of *Ama* and excess *doshas* from the body acts to clear the channels (*srotas*) and tissues (*dhatus*) and make them more receptive to the highly toning, enriching, and rejuvenative herbs and minerals that comprise the elements of rejuvenation therapy. *Rasayana chikitsa* (rejuvenation treatment) is a specialized form of supplementation therapy used in middle and older age to revitalize the tissues and retard the aging process.

THE FIVE PRINCIPAL PROCEDURES OF *PANCHAKARMA* PROPER

Formal (*pradhana*) *Panchakarma* commences only after adequate *Purvakarma* has properly prepared the patient. Inordinate amounts of *Ama* should not be present in the system at this phase of treatment. Although *Ama* is always present to some degree in the body, excessive amounts should have been significantly reduced. Any "loose" *Ama* in the tissues (*dhatus*) and channels (*srotas*) and virtually all *Ama* in the gastrointestinal tract should have been burnt up and eliminated. Vitiated *doshas* that had been embedded in the deep tissues (*shakha*) should now be mobile in order to facilitate their facile movement into the central parts of the body, particularly the entire gastrointestinal tract. In this state of readiness (*utkleshana*), the vitiated *doshas* become accessible and are prepared for subsequent elimination.

Vamana: Therapeutic Emesis

Vamana (therapeutic emesis or vomiting) is the first of the five principal purificatory procedures. Since it is targeted to eliminate vitiated *Kapha*, it is particularly useful in those with *Kapha*-dominant constitutions and in those with *Kapha*-dominant imbalances. The sites of vitiated *Kapha* accumulation are the stomach and the lungs. Such imbalances include but are not restricted to the following: asthma, upper respiratory infections, states of excess phlegm and mucus, i.e., allergies, early stages of diabetes, obesity, migraine, sluggish metabolism, lack of taste sensitivity, and poor appetite. The optimal season for this procedure is spring when *Kapha* is normally provoked by the moist climate. *Vamana* is generally contraindicated in the following situations:

Vata-dominant constitutions; *Vata* imbalances; those under 12 and over 65 years; patients who are emaciated, anorexic, or convalescent; those with upper gastrointestinal or respiratory bleeding, heart disease, ascites, dry cough, constipation, and acute fever.

Vamana is a one-day procedure. It is performed under qualified Ayurvedic supervision, as are all *Panchakarma* treatments. Foods that strongly elicit *Kapha*, such as rice, milk, and yogurt, along with extra salt and sweets are given on the previous day. This diet is called *adhishyandi* (moisture producing) and temporarily increases *Kapha* in the gastrointestinal tract. On the morning of the procedure, the patient is not to eat breakfast although some hot beverage may be taken. Under supervision, he is given about 500 cc or 4 to 8 cups of liquid. This may consist of warm milk with sugar, or a tea of licorice, honey, and salt, or buttermilk and is to be consumed in 15 to 30 minutes. At this point, an emetic herbal preparation that contains calamus, lobelia, or Madana phala (emetic nut) is administered. These are the most commonly used herbs although others may be used depending on the specific situation. In about 45 minutes, vomiting naturally begins; if it does not, some judicious stimulation of the back of the throat with the fingers to activate the gag reflex may trigger vomiting. Vomiting is then guided under close supervision until completion usually within 2 hours.

The vomitus is expelled serially beginning with food substances, then *Kapha*-containing mucus, then yellow-green *Pitta* secretions, and lastly *Vata* gases. Observations and measurement of the expelled contents are made. A quantitative range of the patient's *vamana* is determined. This includes (1) a minimum number (4) of emetic episodes amounting up to about 325 cc; (2) a moderate number (6) of emetic episodes amounting up to 650 cc; and (3) a maximum number (8) resulting in a quantity of vomitus up to 1300 cc.

Adequate or successful *vamana* is reflected in subjective and objective parameters. The patient reports feeling light, uncongested, and relieved; vomiting terminates easily; pre-*Vamana* symptoms are decreased; and the digestive power, experienced as normal appetite, is restored. Inadequate emesis occurs when there is an absence or a very slow onset of vomiting; when only the emetic fluids and herbs are expelled; and when symptoms like a subjective sense of heaviness in the chest and abdomen and lethargy occur; and when signs such as skin rashes appear. The physician supervising the case manages disturbed emetic treatment in a variety of ways.

A definite postemesis regimen is then begun. The basis of this is a very light, graduated food intake (*samsarjana krama)* which occurs over a 3-day period. On day 1, other than intermittent warm and hot liquids such as herbal teas, food intake begins in the evening with *peya*, which is the hot liquid that some Basmati rice has been cooked in without the addition of condiments. On day 2, the morning and afternoon meal consists of *vilepi*, which is a moderate amount of steamed, plain Basmati rice. On the evening of day 2, *akrita yusha*, which is a Basmati rice and yellow split mung dal soup without spices, is consumed. On day 3, the morning and afternoon meal consists of *krita yusha*, which is rice and mung dal soup to which mild spices have been added. On the evening of day 3, a regular diet, proper to the individual's constitutional type, is resumed. Along with the *samsarjana krama* diet, classical Ayurvedic texts recommend several days of rest and the avoidance of any excessive activity as well as exposure to cold both in food and environmentally. In addition, the smoking of medicated, herbal mixtures, devoid of regular tobacco, has been suggested. The *samsarjana krama* concept, in fact, may be the historical precedent for modern postoperative feeding protocols.

Virechana: Therapeutic Purgation

Virechana (therapeutic purgation) is the second of the five principal purificatory procedures. Since it is targeted to eliminate primarily vitiated *Pitta* as well as some *Kapha*, it is particularly useful in those with *Pitta*-dominant constitutions and in those with *Pitta*-dominant imbalances. Vitiated *Pitta* comes out of the liver, gall bladder, spleen, and small intestine and settles in the small intestine. Some *Pitta* imbalances include: skin inflammation, allergic rash, acne, chronic fever, acute diarrhea, the range of hepatic disorders, general inflammatory diseases, and some hematological problems. The aforementioned may and usually do contain some *Kapha* component and *virechana* addresses this aspect as well. As with all *Panchakarma* procedures, *virechana* is used to treat average problems. In the United States, *Panchakarma* is not recommended or used to treat any life-threatening disease, cancer, immune deficiency problem, or terminal illness. The optimal season for *virechana* is summer when *Pitta dosha* is naturally provoked by the hot weather. *Virechana* is generally contraindicated in the following situations: *Vata*-dominant constitutions and *Vata* imbalances; those under 12 and over about 75 years; patients who are emaciated, weak, or who have significant lower gastrointestinal and rectal problems such as bleeding, fissures, chronic diarrhea, and prolapse; menstruating, pregnant, and postpartum women; significant cardiovascular disease; alcoholism; very low *Agni* (digestive capacity); and acute fever.

Virechana is a one-day procedure under Ayurvedic monitoring but able to be done at home outside of a clinic. It is usually performed about 3 days post-*vamana; virechana,* however, may be given as an individual or singular treatment as the case requires. After adequate preparatory oleation and sudation, one may begin *virechana*. Purgation inducing substances are usually administered on an empty stomach the evening before. The selection of an appropriate purgative is varied depending on the individual's specific constitution and condition. Castor oil and senna compounds are commonly used since they are suitable for most situations. For those with *Vata* tendencies, warm milk with ginger or psyllium may be used; for *Pitta* situations, rhubarb, aloe, or psyllium are good choices; for those of *Kapha* constitution, rhubarb, aloe, or Epsom salts work well. Other Ayurvedic herbs and compounds include Haritaki, *Triphala,* Trivrit, and Katuki. Purgation usually begins the next morning and may last until noon. Several bowel movements yielding fecal matter, mucus, and some yellow-colored *Pitta* material are produced. The general character of these is observed and recorded for the physician to assess.

Adequate *virechana* is accompanied by a feeling of lightness in the body and a normal increase in appetite. Inadequate purgation is reflected in the absence of or very little bowel movement, a continued sense of heaviness and discomfort in the abdomen, loss of appetite, and vomiting. In this event, the physician applies appropriate remediation to correct this condition. The post-*virechana* protocol is similar to that for post-*vamana*. It consists of *samsarjana krama* (graduated, light diet) for 3 days and rest; medicated herbal inhalation is not suggested.

Basti: Therapeutic Enema

Basti (therapeutic enema) is the third of the five principal purificatory procedures. It was hailed by Charaka as being the greatest and most efficacious of all treatments. It is useful for all *Vata* imbalances in all constitutional types. *Vata* imbalance manifests in three main areas: (1) neurological disorders; (2) skeletal disorders; and (3) mental disorders. In addition, *basti* is used for chronic constipation, chronic fever, kidney and sexual disorders. The optimal season for *basti* is the fall wherein *Vata* is heavily provoked. Like *virechana, basti* may be done alone and not as part of a *Panchakarma* series. If it is done in series, about 3 days should elapse between the different procedures. *Basti,* considered the safest and simplest of the *Panchakarma* procedures, however, is generally contraindicated in the following: children under 12 years and the elderly over about 75 years; severe emaciation; diarrhea; diabetes; acute fever; anemia; asthma; vomiting; chronic poor digestion, especially accompanied by excess *Kapha* and *Ama* in the gastrointestinal tract; and liver disorders with ascites.

Basti occurs within a 24-hour period. It may be done at home or in a clinic under supervision. Preparation includes only external oleation, sudation, and no intake of food 6 hours before the procedure. There are many types and subtypes of *basti.* The two most common are (1) *niruha-asthapana* (herbal cleansing decoction); and (2) *anuvasana* (oil retention). The composition of the *niruha-asthapana basti* may vary considerably. A common formulation consists of about 200 cc of sesame oil, 250 cc of an herbal decoction that may include the *dashmoola* compound (10 Ayurvedic herbs), calamus, fennel, ginger, and some salt. This amounts to about 16 ounces or 2 cups of liquid. It is administered, per rectum, either early in the morning or in late afternoon, and retained for at least 15 minutes and up to 50 minutes. It is then evacuated and the procedure is terminated. The *anuvasana basti,* unlike the *niruha-asthapana basti,* is less cleansing but more tonifying and nourishing. Its composition is made up primarily of sesame oil (2 to 4 ounces) with some warm water, salt, and, perhaps, a small amount of a mild decoction of toning herbs. The *anuvasana basti* is administered at bedtime, retained overnight, and then evacuated in the morning.

A relatively complete bowel evacuation, a sense of relief and well-being, and a normalized appetite follow adequate *basti.* Inadequate *basti* is an uncommon occurrence. A post-*basti* regimen is lenient and includes recommendations for rest and light diet.

Nasya: Intranasal Therapy

Nasya (intranasal therapy) is one of the last of the five principal purificatory procedures. It is indicated in the treatment of any or all of the *doshas* that are situated in the head and neck region. In this way, it is less targeted and broader in range covering treatment of the five senses, including the throat, the nasal passages, and aspects of the brain or central nervous system. The importance of *nasya* therapy is reflected in the ancient saying: "*Nasa hi shiraso dwarum*" meaning the nose is the doorway to the contents of the head. This connotes the possibility of affecting the subtle or energetic dimensions of the individual including breathing, *Prana* (vital energy), mental functioning, and consciousness.

There are several types of *nasya.* Some of these include the following.

1. *Pradhamana-virechana nasya,* cleansing *nasya.* This is performed using dry herbal powders, such as Brahmi, ginger, sage, or calamus, which are inhaled. This cleansing treatment specifically reduces excess *Kapha* in the head area.
2. *Bruhana nasya,* nutritional *nasya.* This is performed using oils such as ghee or sesame with the addition of nourishing herbs

such as ashwaghanda, shatavari, or tulsi. *Vata* imbalances in the head area, such as migraines, anxiety, and agitation, for example, are responsive to this treatment.

3. *Shamana nasya,* palliative *nasya.* Medicated oils and herbal decoctions are applied intranasally to reduce aggravated *Pitta* disorders as, for example, conjunctivitis, tinnitus, and even hair loss.
4. *Navana nasya,* oil and herbal decoction *nasya.* This is useful in mixed *Vata-Pitta* and in mixed *Kapha-Pitta* disorders.
5. *Marshya nasya,* strong purificatory *nasya.* This refers to a large quantity (8 to 32 drops) of medicinal substance applied intranasally.
6. *Pratimarshya,* mild palliative *nasya.* This refers to a very small (2 drops per nostril) amount of medicinal substance used intranasally. This form of *nasya* is recommended for everyone as an aid to daily health maintenance. It usually consists of a small amount of plain ghee or of plain or herbalized sesame oil put on the pinky finger and gently inserted in each nostril using mild lubricating and massaging motion.
7. *Dhooma nasya,* inhalation or smoking of dry herbs. This *nasya* is used after *vamana* since it, like *vamana,* dispels *Kapha.* It is also part of the post-*Panchakarma* protocol. Herbs such as cloves, calamus, and bayberry are used. Tobacco is never used.

Nasya can be used alone or as part of a classical *Panchakarma* routine in which case it would follow any of the other procedures with an interval of 1 to 2 days. Before and after *nasya,* mild oleation and sudation to the face, throat, and neck are recommended. At the completion of the procedure, a small amount of ghee is applied intranasally.

***Raktamoksha*: Therapeutic Blood Purification**

Raktamoksha (therapeutic blood purification) is the last principal procedure of classical *Panchakarma.* As was mentioned earlier, it was devised in ancient times by the Ayurvedic surgeon, Sushruta (c. 660 B.C.), who regarded it as highly efficacious. He laid such great emphasis on *rakta dhatu* (blood tissue) that he considered it to be the fourth *dosha*. The quality of blood, its purity, and its impure states, is a leading concern in Ayurveda. Since *Pitta dosha* is the product of the breakdown of blood (*rakta mala*), blood and the condition of *Pitta* are closely intertwined. In addition, the body's digestive fire (*Agni)* uses *Pitta dosha* as its vehicle and modus operandi.

Raktamoksha is a therapeutic intervention considered in some cases of *Pitta* and blood vitiation. Such conditions include the following: skin infections, skin inflammations, urticaria, rashes, acne, eczema, hives, gout, some hematological, hepatic, and splenic disorders. Some major contraindications include anemia, severe emaciation, edema, menstruation, pregnancy, asthma, impotency, and in the very young (under 12 years) and the elderly (over 75 years).

Classical Ayurveda has distinguished several types of *raktamoksha*. Some of the most important are the following.

1. *Prachhana,* blood letting using quick, sharp incisions.
2. *Siravyadha,* removal of blood by syringe.
3. *Jalauka,* the use of topically applied leeches. This classical method is considered the mildest and one of the most effective. It, like the other bloodletting techniques, is still used in India under medical supervision.

Therapeutic bloodletting is not performed in the United States; other, less invasive, means have been devised to address what are considered impure or toxic blood conditions. These methods use herbal substances that specifically target impurities in the blood. Herbs that are primarily bitter and those with some astringent characteristics, such as burdock root, katuki, turmeric, goldenseal, pomegranate, and neem have been used. These herbal interventions are coupled with restrictions of *Pitta*-aggravating dietary substances such as yogurt, salt, sour and fermented items (citrus, soy sauce), vinegar, and alcohol.

UTTARAKARMA: POST-*PANCHAKARMA* REGIMEN

When a course of *Panchakarma* is completed, *Uttarakarma,* also called *Paschatakarma* (follow-up actions), is prescribed. These include both dietary and lifestyle recommendations that facilitate the gradual reentry of the newly treated person back into a regular, daily routine. The intensity of the entire purificatory experience alters the intrinsic state of the tissues and the metabolism. Large amounts of *Ama* and vitiated *doshas* have thus been eliminated with an opening of the channels and cleansing of the tissues resulting from this physiological debridement. The tissues, therefore, are purified and in a state of enhanced receptivity. A mild and graduated diet, along with selected toning herbs, helps restore their nutrition and strength. In addition, clinical experience has demonstrated that the overall condition of the *Agni* is greatly reduced following the purificatory procedures. This temporarily lowered state must be clearly recognized and addressed with the *samsarjana krama* (graduated diet) suggestions. The classical dietary regimen is as follows.

1. *Manda,* rice water. This is the plain broth in which Basmati rice has been cooked. A small amount of ghee and saindhava (Indian rock salt) or Indian black salt and ghee are added.
2. *Peya,* thin rice soup. This is a very thin mixture of Basmati rice cooked in about 8 parts of water with some salt and ghee.
3. *Vilepi,* thick rice soup. This is Basmati rice cooked with about 4 parts of water to which a very small amount of salt, ghee, and mild herbs such as ginger, fennel, turmeric, cumin, and coriander have been added.
4. *Odana,* plain cooked rice.
5. *Yusha,* light soup. This is a mixture of Basmati rice and a small amount of split yellow mung dal (lentils) cooked together in a manner similar to *vilepi.*
6. *Kichari.* This is a more substantial mixture of Basmati rice and split yellow mung dal cooked with spices and vegetables.

Although the time frames may vary according to the constitution and condition of the individual patient, the above *samsarjana krama* is observed over the course of about 3 days. On day 1, only *manda* and *peya* are consumed; on day 2, *vilepi* and *odana;* and on day 3, *yusha* as the first meal, and *kichari* as the evening meal. After this, a regular diet according to one's *prakruti* (constitutional body type) is resumed. Overeating is to be avoided at all times.

Daily routines should resume in a graduated fashion over the course of about 1 week. Inordinate physical activity and exposure to cold both dietary and environmental should be avoided.

APPENDIX 1

AYURVEDIC ORAL AND WRITTEN TRADITION TIMELINE

These works have only approximate dates of origin and many are not available in English translation.

Pre-1000 B.C.: Vedic *rishis* receive and transmit the Ayurvedic conception as an oral tradition that only later becomes explicitly codified in the four Vedic texts, *Rig-Veda, Sama-Veda, Yajur-Veda,* and especially the *Athara-Veda.*

c. 760 B.C.: *Charaka Samhita* of Charaka. This is the axiomatic, foundational text, broadest in scope, that delineates Ayurvedic medicine.

c. 660 B.C.: *Sushruta Samhita* of Sushruta. This is the next fundamental medical text but with a strong emphasis on the structure, functioning, and treatment of blood tissue and on surgery.

c. A.D. 100: Nagarjuna's texts on Materia Medica with original contributions of iatrochemistry, the medicinal preparation of minerals.

c. A.D. seventh century: *Ashtanga Sagraha* and *Ashtanga Hridaya* of Vagbhata of Sind: texts that are a summary of the previous works of Charaka and Sushruta.

c. 1331: *Madhava Nidana* of Madhava (Vidyaraya) of Kishkindha, southern India. This is the most comprehensive text that delineates Ayurvedic diagnosis and the classification of disease.

c. 14th century: *Sarangadhara Samhita.* Ayurvedic pulse diagnosis presented in detail.

c. 1483: *Rasapradipa* by Vashaldeva. This text describes the medicinal use of purified mercury preparations.

c. 1495: *Rasamrita* by Pandit Vaidya Kendra. This work describes the pharmacology of mineral and metal medicinal substances.

c. 1550: *Bhavaprakasha* by Bhava Mishra of Madra Desha near Benares in northwest India. This is held to be the most important summary of the scope of all Ayurvedic medicine to date with special attention to dietary and rejuvenative treatment innovations.

c. 1633: *Yogaratnakara* by Nayanashekara, a Jain priest. This text elaborates the art of compounding medicinal preparations.

c. 1734: *Ayurveda Prakasha* by Madhava of Benares. This is a work on Materia Medica.

c. 1751: *Yogatarangini* by Trimulla Bhatta: a nosology of Ayurvedic Materia Medica.

c. 1794: *Jvaraparajaya* by Jayaravi: a work on the nature of fever.

c. 1859: *Hastamalka* by Bavabhai. This is an updated consideration of the preparation of mineral-based medicinal preparations.

c. 1867: *Nighantaratnakara* by Vishnu Vasudeva Godbole. The body of this work constitutes additional notes on Ayurvedic medicine and pharmacology.

APPENDIX 2

DISEASES CAUSED BY THE *DOSHAS*

DISORDERS CAUSED BY *VATA*

1. *Nakhabheda* (cracking of nails)
2. *Vipadika* (cracking, sores, or blisters of feet)
3. *Padasula* (pain in foot)
4. *Padabhramsa* (peroneal nerve palsy)
5. *Padasuptata* (numbness of foot)
6. *Vatakhuddata* (club and painful foot)
7. *Gulphagraha* (stiff and painful ankle)
8. *Pindikodvestana* (calf cramps)
9. *Gridhrasi* (sciatica)
10. *Janubheda* (bow legs)
11. *Januvislesa* (knock knees)
12. *Urustambha* (stiffness, arthritis, or paralysis of thigh)
13. *Urusada* (thigh pain and weakness)
14. *Pangulya* (paraplegia)
15. *Gudabhramsa* (prolapsed rectum)
16. *Gudarti* (tenesmus or rectal ulceration)
17. *Vrisanaksepa* (pain or hernia in scrotum)
18. *Sephastambha* (stiffness of penis)
19. *Vanksananaha* (pain and tenseness in groin)
20. *Sronibheda* or *Conitabheda* (pain, possibly bleeding, around the pelvic girdle)
21. *Vidbheda* (diarrhea)
22. *Udavarta* (peristaltic dysfunction)
23. *Khanjatva* (ambulation disorder)
24. *Kubjatva* (kyphosis)
25. *Vamanatva* (dwarfism)
26. *Trikagraha* (arthritis of sacroiliac joint)

27. *Pristhagraha* (stiffness and pain in the back)
28. *Parsvavamarda* (pain in chest or flanks)
29. *Udaravesta* (spasmodic abdominal pain)
30. *Hrinmoha* (bradycardia)
31. *Hriddrava* (tachycardia)
32. *Vaksa Uddharsa* (dull chest pain felt as coming from inside)
33. *Vaksa Uparodha* (impairment of thoracic movement felt as imposed from outside)
34. *Vaksastoda* (stabbing pain in chest)
35. *Bahusosa* (atrophy of arm)
36. *Grivastambha* (stiffness of neck)
37. *Manyastambha* (torticollis)
38. *Kanthoddhvamsa* (hoarseness)
39. *Hanubheda* (jaw pain, dislocation of face bones)
40. *Osthabheda* (lip pain)
41. *Aksibheda* (eye pain)
42. *Dantabheda* (toothache or tooth loss)
43. *Dantasathilya* (loose teeth)
44. *Mukatva* (aphasia)
45. *Vaksanga* (hesitant, stammering speech)
46. *Kasayasyata* (astringent taste in mouth)
47. *Mukhasosa* (dry mouth)
48. *Arasajnata* (impairment of taste)
49. *Ghrananasa* (impairment of smell)
50. *Karnasula* (earache)
51. *Asabdasravana* (tinnitus and partial hearing loss)
52. *Uccaihsriti* (hard of hearing)
53. *Badhirya* (deafness)
54. *Vartmastambha* (ptosis or paralysis of eyelid)
55. *Vartmasankoca* (eyelid inversion)
56. *Timira* (cataract)
57. *Aksisula* (pinching pain in eye)
58. *Aksivyudasa* (ptosis of eyeball)
59. *Sankhabheda* (pain fracture in temporal skull bone)
60. *Bhruvyudasa* (ptosis of eyebrow)
61. *Lalatabheda* (pain or fracture in frontal skull bone)
62. *Siroruk* (headache)
63. *Kesabhumisphutana* (dandruff or scalp sores)
64. *Ardita* (facial paralysis)

65. *Ekangaroga* (monoplegia)
66. *Sarvangaroga* (polyplegia)
67. *Paksavadha* (hemiplegia)
68. *Aksepaka* (clonic convulsion)
69. *Dandaka* (tonic convulsion)
70. *Tama* (severe fatigue or fainting)
71. *Bhrama* (giddiness or dizziness)
72. *Yepathu* (tremor)
73. *Jirmbha* (yawning)
74. *Hikka* (hiccup)
75. *Visada* (asthenia)
76. *Atipralapa* (delirium)
77. *Rauksa Parusya* (dryness and hardness)
78. *Syavarunavabhasata* (dusky red complexion)
79. *Asvapna* or *Asapna* (insomnia)
80. *Anavasthitacittatva* (mental disorder and agitation)

DISORDERS CAUSED BY *PITTA*

1. *Osa* (sensation of inordinate body heat)
2. *Plosa* (sensation of body being scorched by fire)
3. *Daha* (sensation of burning)
4. *Davathu* (sensation of boiling)
5. *Dhumaka* (sensation of fuming)
6. *Amlaka* (acid eructation)
7. *Vidaha* (burning sensation in the chest)
8. *Antardaha* (burning sensation in the chest)
9. *Amsadaha* (burning sensation in the shoulders)
10. *Usmadhikya* (increased temperature)
11. *Atisveda* (excessive perspiration)
12. *Angagandha* (unpleasant body odor)
13. *Angavadarana* (cracking pain or sores on the body)
14. *Sonitakleda* (hematological disorder)
15. *Mamsakleda* (muscular disorder)
16. *Tvagdaha* (burning sensation of the skin)
17. *Tvagavadarana* (cracking of the skin)
18. *Carmadalana* (itching of the skin)
19. *Raktakostha* (urticaria)

20. *Raktavisphota* (red vesicles)
21. *Raktapitta* (bleeding tendency)
22. *Raktamandala* (red wheals)
23. *Haritatva* (green tinge to the skin)
24. *Haridratva* (yellow tinge to the skin)
25. *Nilika* (blue or black skin moles)
26. *Kaksa* (herpes or skin abscesses)
27. *Kamala* (jaundice)
28. *Tiktasyata* (bitter taste in the mouth)
29. *Lohitagandhasyata* (smell of blood from the mouth)
30. *Putimukhata* (halitosis)
31. *Trisnadhikya* (excessive thirst)
32. *Atripti* (inability to feel satiated)
33. *Asyavipaka* (stomatitis)
34. *Galapaka* (pharyngitis)
35. *Aksipaka* (conjunctivitis)
36. *Gudapaka* (proctitis)
37. *Medhrapaka* (inflammation of the penis)
38. *Jivadana* (bloody stools)
39. *Tamahpravesa* (delirium and fainting)
40. *Haritaharida netra muttra varcastva* (greenish and yellowish coloration of eyes, urine, and feces)

DISORDERS CAUSED BY *KAPHA*

1. *Tripti* (the sense of feeling full without having eaten)
2. *Tandra* (drowsiness)
3. *Nidradhikya* (excessive sleep)
4. *Staimitya* (timidity)
5. *Gurugatrata* (heaviness of the body)
6. *Alasya* (lethargy)
7. *Mukhamadhurya* (sweet taste in the mouth)
8. *Mukhasrava* (salivation)
9. *Slesmodgirana* (mucus expectoration)
10. *Maladhikya* (excessive excretion of bodily wastes)
11. *Balasada* (severe loss of strength)
12. *Apakti* (inability to digest food)
13. *Hridayopalepa* (fluid buildup in the cardiac region)

14. *Kanthopalepa* (phlegm adhering to the throat)
15. *Dhamanipraticaya* (hardening of vessels)
16. *Galaganda* (goiter)
17. *Atisthaulya* (obesity)
18. *Sitagnitva* (suppression of digestive power and loss of appetite)
19. *Udarda* (uticaria or erysipelas)
20. *Svetavabhasata* and *Svetamutranetravarcastva* (pallor and whiteness of urine, eye, and feces)

APPENDIX 3

CLINICAL CASE EXAMPLES

The following is a representative sampling of some common disorders. The views of Western medicine and those of Ayurveda are compared. Standard medical treatments of disease and Ayurvedic approaches toward balancing vitiated *doshas* are presented. The perspective put forth here is one of offering treatment choices and, perhaps, mutually enhancing, complementary treatment strategies. Illness manifestations are unique in each patient. In Ayurveda, the orienting principles of assessment and management rest on the detailed analysis of *Vata, Pitta,* and *Kapha.* The careful evaluation of *prakruti* (individual constitution) is given punctilious attention. Nuances of the manifold qualities and attributes of the *doshas,* and the specific circumstances of timing, lifecycle stage, and the seasons play a significant role in the inception and manifestation of the disease process, all of which impacts the quality of the patient's life. A rational approach to any disorder would include an appropriate examination by a qualified medical doctor in order to secure a sound diagnosis and treatment plan. This then provides one with a rational basis for the selection of appropriate and reasonable treatment choices. The following examples of Ayurvedically based care represent commonly seen, broad clinical presentations, and are submitted, in general terms, only to suggest general management guidelines. Therapies that are more specific must be individualized by the medical doctor or the Ayurvedic practitioner depending on the particular manifestations of a disorder as it emerges at a particular time in the life of a patient. An important therapeutic issue and difference between Western medicine and Ayurvedic approaches is that Ayurveda addresses developing trends (imbalances of the *doshas*) that, if left unchecked, may develop into fully manifested disorders. In addition, Ayurveda always takes into consideration the complete biopsychospiritual person when assessing and recommending balancing approaches. The comprehensive nature of Ayurvedic evaluation and care incorporating both physical and psychological aspects (*umada*) can even be found in the writings of Charaka over 2,000 years ago (Haldipur, 1984, 1989).

PREMENSTRUAL SYNDROME

Premenstrual syndrome (PMS) is a recurrent condition that affects about 35% of menstruating women with peak occurrences in the 30's and 40's. The clinical presentation manifests about 7 to 14 days before the onset of menstruation. While the signs and symptoms may be varied, the following are often present: decreased energy level, irritability, mood sensitivity, tension, general malaise, dysphoria, altered libido, breast pain, backache, abdominal bloating, and edematous swelling of hands and ankles. The biological mechanisms responsible for PMS are complex. Some major features, however, include relatively high estrogen and relatively low progesterone levels with an increased ratio of estrogen to progesterone; corpus luteum insufficiency with increased prolactin levels; and possibly lowered thyroid function and elevated cortisol levels.

While Western medicine recognizes the occurrence of this syndrome, there is no consensus regarding formal and standardized treatment. Symptoms such as pain are treated with analgesic medications, depression with antidepressants, and edema with antidiuretic drugs, for example. Ayurveda approaches the treatment of PMS by first examining the individual patient to establish the basic *prakruti* (constitutional type), and then the *vikruti* (current state of *dosha* imbalance within the *prakruti*). Although all three *doshas* (*Vata, Pitta,* and *Kapha*) may be vitiated, *Vata* is usually the primary *dosha* with *Pitta* and *Kapha* being secondarily affected.

Treatment strategies address each *dosha*. *Kapha* is usually increased due to excess *Ama* (toxins). This results in edema, sluggishness, and lowered energy level. Dietary recommendations would include a lighter than average diet and the avoidance of all cold foods and dairy products. Hot tea and ample amounts of dry and fresh ginger in tea and foods would act to reduce excess *Kapha* and *Ama*. This, in turn, would reduce the associated signs and symptoms. The vitiated *Pitta* aspects of PMS show as irritability, mood sensitivity, sensations of heat, skin irritation, and irregular menstrual blood flow. To the extent that this may be the dominant clinical presentation, one would recommend an anti-*Pitta* diet that would exclude meat, nuts, alcohol, sour fruits, fermented foods, hot spices, and include more cooling foods like small amounts of dairy products, ghee, vegetables, and salads. Herbs such as aloe vera, turmeric, coriander, fennel, and saffron could be added to foods. The *Vata* aspect of PMS presents as anxiety, depression, insomnia, constipation, and cramping. To the extent that these symptoms predominate, one would recommend a diet that is warm, moderately oily, and regular as opposed to light or heavy. Herbs that balance *Vata* include shatavari, cinnamon, licorice, asafetida, and nutmeg. *Abhyanga* (oil massage) with warm sesame oil is particularly beneficial to pacify vitiated *Vata* and reduce dysphoria and agitation; the use of warm castor oil packs on the lower abdomen may also be soothing.

ATTENTION-DEFICIT/HYPERACTIVITY DISORDER

Attention-Deficit / Hyperactivity Disorder (ADHD) is a disruptive behavior disorder usually beginning in childhood before age 7 (Ninivaggi, 1999). Poor attention and concentration, motoric overactivity, and impulsivity characterize its presentation. Poor organizational skills, academic difficulties, low self-esteem, and behavioral problems often accompany this symptom constellation and manifest both at home and at school. Up to 5 % of the school-age population is affected, with a preponderance of boys. ADHD usually occurs in conjunction with other psychiatric disorders and may be a secondary feature of or may disguise a primary problem such as a major mood disorder or a posttraumatic stress experience. There are no medically established causes responsible for producing this condition. Psychiatry considers it a clinical diagnosis with a variety of mixed, contributing etiologies.

Western medicine treats ADHD with combined psychopharmacological and psychosocial interventions. Often, the psychostimulant drugs, such as methylphenidate, dextroamphetamine, and Adderall, are used. These substances are tightly controlled by the Drug Enforcement Agency of the federal government because of their abuse potential, tolerance, and withdrawal liabilities. As with all medications, there may be undesirable adverse drug effects. Other medications may be used, especially to address the other target symptoms that often accompany ADHD. The range of psychotherapies includes individual, group, and family therapy as well as a variety of behavior management strategies. Specialized educational programming is always necessary. Since the condition is usually chronic, treatments may go on for years.

Ayurveda considers ADHD to be a primary disorder of *Vata*. Treatment, therefore, includes a strict *Vata*-pacifying protocol. Some important features of this are the following. In general, nurturing, warming, moistening, calming, and grounding qualities should characterize all interventions. Dietary guidelines would stress a substantive, nutritive, and wholesome diet that predominates in tastes that are sweet, sour, and salty. Since food allergies play some role in health and disease, a diet that minimizes dairy and wheat products, and emphasizes rice, oats, fish, chicken, eggs, nuts, seeds, cooked vegetables, sweet and some citrus fruits, and oils is recommended. Most beans, raw vegetables, dry fruits, dry light snacks such as popcorn, and soda should be avoided. Food spices that are moderate in nature, such as ginger, fennel, cardamom, and cinnamon, may be used to optimize digestion. There are a variety of herbal tonics, such as ashwaghanda, shatavari, jatamansi, gotu kola, and basil, for example, that may be used depending on the needs of the patient. Modified *abhyanga* (oil massage) is of great benefit. Small amounts of oils such as sesame and almond may be gently massaged on parts of the head and feet before bed. Lifestyle suggestions would include early rising by 7 to 8 A.M., going to sleep about 10 P.M., and the reduction and significant moderation of highly stimulating activities such as listening to loud music, excessive watching of TV and movies, and excessive physical exercise.

A program of guided quiet time, i.e., meditation and breathing regulation (*pranayama*), should be structured into the child's daily routine by a responsible adult. As mentioned in Chapter 9, aspects of Yoga techniques, especially those directed to self-regulation of the body (*Hatha* Yoga) and the mind (*dhyana*) may contribute to increased attention and concentration. The quality time that a parent spends with a child may be viewed as therapeutic in the broadest sense; its therapeutic value is inestimable. One would consider, of course, the mutually enhancing interventions of the appropriate psychotherapies and solid educational programming to complement Ayurvedic care.

ASTHMA

Asthma is a disease of the respiratory airways characterized by inflammation, increased responsiveness of the tracheobronchial tree to a multiplicity of stimuli, neuronal activation, changes in vascular permeability, and increased mucus production. Signs and symptoms of narrowing of the air passages include paroxysms of shortness of breath, cough, and wheezing. This takes an episodic course with acute exacerbations being interspersed with periods of remission.

Western medicine regards the etiology of the spectrum of asthmatic presentations as heterogeneous and ambiguous at this time although the inflammatory process is central. Subtypes are classified by the principal stimuli that trigger a flare-up. This distinction is regarded as artificial, in part, since specific causative factors and clear-cut disease states continue to be under investigation in order to refine current views. Three broad subtypes are recognized: (1) extrinsic or atopic asthma that has an allergic component characterized by elevated levels of serum IgE, the allergic antibody, and a personal or family history of asthma; (2) intrinsic or idiosyncratic asthma that appears not due to allergy and not having a family history, but rather the result of factors such as toxic chemicals, infection, exercise, cold air, and emotional stressors; and (3) mixed group asthma that has features of both the aforementioned types. Approximately 4 to 5% of the U.S. population is affected, and children under 10 constitute about 50% of cases. A commonly used four step classification of asthma severity is based on clinical features before treatment. Step 1 is mild and intermittent asthma; step 2 is mild and persistent; step 3 is moderate and persistent; and step 4 is severe and persistent.

Since an asthmatic attack may become a medical emergency, only a qualified medical doctor should evaluate and treat this potentially life-threatening circumstance. Routine care, according to Western medicine, includes attempts at removing known and suspected environmental causes, e.g., allergens, house dust, mold, fungi, and smoke, as well as using additional preventative desensitization or immunotherapy. Drug treatments are commonly used to control asthma. Chronic management includes: (1) drugs that inhibit smooth muscle contraction, i.e., specific inhaler broncodilators, especially for acute exacerbations; (2) agents that prevent or reverse inflammation such as glucocorticoids and mast cell-stabilizing agents, especially for chronic maintenance; and (3) drugs that have antihistaminic and decongestant properties only as medically prescribed according to the needs of the particular condition. Ongoing medical monitoring care is mandatory.

Svasa roga or asthma is a condition that has been recognized in Ayurveda for thousands of years. Five types have been classified: (1) *maha svasa*, or great asthma, is the most severe and may include what in the West is called "status asthmaticus"; (2) *urdhva svasa*, or upwards asthma, a serious condition characterized by great difficulty in inhalation; (3) *chinna svasa*, or broken asthma, characterized by very irregular breathing that periodically halts, distension of the abdomen, and possible hemorrhaging in the head area; (4) *tamaka svasa*, or allergic asthma, characterized by pain, dryness, and wheezing; and (5) *ksudra svasa*, or minor asthma, characterized by minor and transient asthmatic symptomatology.

In Ayurvedic theory, all asthma components originate in the stomach, then pass though the channels carrying *rasa* (plasma) until they finally localize in the lungs. After comprehensive evaluation and assessment to determine the specifics of the particular case, interventions always begin by correcting the *Kapha* imbalances in the stomach. Since acute exacerbations may be life threatening, they should be treated by conventional medical techniques. Preventative care, i.e., between attacks, is conducive to Ayurvedic prophylaxis.

To prevent and reduce inordinate production of mucus, a *Kapha*-pacifying diet would include avoidance of all dairy products, no cold foods, and the inclusion of a light diet of cooked vegetables with as many pungent food spices (black pepper, red pepper, sage, ginger, etc.) as is possible to consume comfortably. Yogurt and bananas are to be avoided since they strongly increase *Kapha*. The therapeutic herb, pippali, is very useful in resolving vitiated *Kapha* conditions. When *Pitta* vitiation, evidenced by the production of yellow mucus, inflammation, and irritation, is prominent, then *Pitta*-pacifying herbs are added. These may include coriander, gotu kola, and turmeric. In addition to *Kapha* and *Pitta* factors, there is always a disturbance of *Vata* manifested by increased motoric activity and agitation. When this is an outstanding feature of the clinical presentation, a *Vata*-pacifying diet, recommendations for a slower paced lifestyle, and herbs such as haritaki, asafetida, and a mineral-based preparation of mica called *abhraka bhasma* are given. Respiratory distress is aggravated by the improper upward movement of *Apana Vata;* the aforementioned diet, herbs, and minerals tend to normalize this. In addition, moist heat with aromatic herbs and oils such as eucalyptus and menthol applied to the chest helps to liquefy excess *Kapha* and aid in relaxing and opening bronchial airways.

GLOSSARY

Abhraka bhasma: Ayurvedically prepared mineral-based medicine with mica as the principal ingredient.

Abhyanga: Whole body oil massage.

Abyantar: Therapeutic internal oleation treatment.

Adana Kala: The hot and dry time of the year; generally summer in the United States; see AGNEYA.

Adana: Plain cooked rice.

Adhishyandi: Therapeutic and moistening diet used to increase vitiated *doshas* on a temporary basis.

Adhyatmika: Causes of a disease that originate from within the physical body: (1) *adhibala* (genetic); (2) *janmaja* (congenital); and (3) *dosaja* (due to *doshas*).

Adhibhautika: Causes of a disease that originate in the external environment.

Adhidaivika: Causes of a disease that have more esoteric origins, i.e., *karma,* fate, etc.

Advaita: Nonduality.

Advaita Vedanta: The *darshana* or worldview made explicit by Shankara (ninth century A.D.) stressing the absolute unity of all reality; also called *Utarra Mimamsa.*

Agadatantra: Toxicology, one of the eight branches of Ayurveda.

Agantu: Exogenous causes of disease.

Agneya: The warm and hot time of the year; in the United States, usually spring and summer.

Agni: Fire. In the Vedas: *Agni* is personified as a deity; both the deity and the physical, externally real fire that is the centerpiece of the most sacred ritual observance. In Ayurveda, *Agni* is the internal digestive fire responsible for nutrient transformation and tissue and cellular assimilation.

Agnimandya: Impaired *Agni.*

Ahamkara: The individualized ego or circumscribed identity of any biological being.

Ahara rasa: The preliminary state of the nutritive fluid just after ingestion and before primary digestion has begun.

Aharayogin: Spices.

Ahimsa: Nonviolence.

Ajna Chakra: The sixth energy node along the *sushumna* or central energy channel located in the area of the brain between the eyes.

Akasha: The Ether or Space great Element.

Akrita yusha: Mixture of rice and mung lentils in mild soup base.

Alochaka Pitta: The subdosha of *Pitta* associated with vision in the eyes.

Ama: The toxic metabolic end product resulting from improper digestion; one of several factors that contributes to disease.

Amalaki: Amla fruit *(Emblica officinalis).*

Amaya: Disease.

Ambu: Water.

Amla: Sour taste; *Amla* medicinal fruit (*Emblica officinalis).*

Amrit: Nectar.

Anabolism: The metabolic phase of cellular and tissue buildup.

Anahata Chakra: The energy node located in the region of the heart.

Ananda: Bliss.

Anandamaya Kosha: The bliss sheath; the last of five layers or sheaths that compose the individual human being.

Anguli pramana: Bodily proportions.

Anna: Food.

Annamaya Kosha: The food sheath; the gross, physical body; the first of five layers or sheaths and the most material dimension comprising the complete individual.

Annapanavidhi: Nutrition.

Annavaha Srotas: The digestive system, alimentary canal, or gastrointestinal tract.

Antahkarana: The inner organ or instrument of cognition and feeling; also *Antarindriya;* includes *Buddhi, Ahamkara,* and *Manas.*

Antarindriya: Antahkarana.

Antar Marga: The inner disease pathway consisting of the gastrointestinal canal.

Antharmarga: The gastrointestinal tract.

Anubhava: Awareness that develops from a surface understanding toward a more direct, intuitive, and profound apprehension.

Anumana: Reasoning based on inference.

Anuvasana Basti: Therapeutic enema of oil and herbs.

Ap: One of the five great gross Elements, Water; also *Jala, Apas.*

Apana Vata: The downward moving subdosha of *Vata* primarily located in the colon.

Aparigraha: Nonoverindulgence.

Apas: The Element of Water; also called *Jala, Ap.*

Apta: The inspired and authoritative wisdom of sages (*rishis*).

Aptopadesha/Shabda: Information from texts, authoritative literature, and interviews.

Aranyakas: Texts of the Vedas composed in the forests and that consist of mystical interpretations of the chronologically earlier Vedic teachings.

Aristha: Herbal wine; connotation of an omen, sign, or symptom with a negative prognosis.

Arogya: Health.

Artav: Menstrual fluid; also spelled *artava.*

Artav Beej: Maternal genetic material.

Artavavaha Srotas: The menstrual system.

Artha: Necessary and appropriate material wealth; the Vedic life goal of securing appropriate wealth and possessions; also meaning the objects possessed by the five senses.

Arunasayava: Skin discolorations.

Aryavarta: Ancient Vedic name for present day India.

Asadhya: Disease with an unfavorable prognosis.

Asafetida: Spice (*Ferula asafoetida*).

Asamkara: Unprocessed.

Asana: Yoga posture.

Asantarpana: The difficult and arduous psychological sense that one experiences when undergoing *langhana* or reducing therapies that require abstinence.
Asatmya: Unwholesome.
Asatmyendryartha Samyoga: The unwholesome and incompatible contact of the sense organs with their objects; this can range from no contact to excessive contact; a fundamental factor in the universal etiology of all disorders.
Ashaya: Hollow viscera.
Ashtavidha Pariksha: The diagnostic examination of a patient using 8 parameters.
Ashwaghanda: Herbal root (*Withania somnifera)*.
Asmita: Unhealthy egoism.
Asrama: The Vedic delineation of four stages of life: student, family life, self-inquiry, and active pursuit of *moksha*.
Asteya: Nonstealing.
Asthanga: Eight limbs.
Asthanga Ayurveda: The eight branches of Ayurvedic medicine: (1) internal medicine; (2) surgery; (3) otolaryngology and ophthalmology; (4) obstetrics, gynecology, and pediatrics; (5) toxicology; (6) psychiatry; (7) antiaging medicine; and (8) reproductive and aphrodisiac medicine.
Asthanga Hridaya: Ayurvedic text written by the Ayurvedic surgeon, Vagbhata (c. seventh century A.D.).
Asthi: Bone tissue.
Asthidhara kala: The membrane of bone; also the membrane of the colon.
Asthivaha Srotas: The channels of circulation of bone tissue.
Astika darshana: Any orthodox worldview based on the primary authority of the Vedas.
Atapa-sevana: Therapeutic sun bathing.
Athara-Veda: One of the four primary Vedas, considered the last one compiled, that is composed of 731 hymns whose content includes atonement ceremonies, maledictions, marriage and burial songs, and medical formulas.
Atman: The real, immortal Self or spirit of an individual; the microcosmic correlate of *Brahman*.
Aura: The subtle energy field emanating from the body.
Aushada: Herb or drug; also *oshadhi*.

Avalambaka Kapha: The subdosha of *Kapha* providing lubrication in the chest and spine.

Avaleha: Herbal formula with the consistency of a jelly or jam.

Avasthamabhana: Support, especially of the colon provided by the feces.

Avasthapaka: Primary digestion; also *prapaka.*

Avidya: Ignorance.

Avyakta: Pure existence in its unmanifest state.

Ayurveda: The knowledge, science, and wisdom of life and longevity; an *Upaveda* or accessory Veda to the *Athara-Veda.*

Ayu: Life.

Ayus: Life; a period or measure of life; see *Ayu.*

Ayushah pramana: Lifespan as the quantitative measure of an individual's duration of life.

Bala: Strength or power in the body; childhood; the herb *Sida cordifolia.*

Bahya: Therapeutic external oil massage.

Bahya Marga: The outer disease pathway consisting of the skin and the blood.

Bandha: Bondage to or dependence on the material world that is mediated by the sensory faculties.

Bandhu: Correspondence or harmonizing, meaningful link between ritual, lifestyle routines, and the cosmic order.

Basil: Herb (*Ocinum spp).*

Basti: Ayurvedic therapeutic enema.

Bayamarga: The disease pathways leading into the limbs and deeper tissues.

Bhagavad Gita: The sixth book of the Indian national epic poem, *Mahabharata,* composed between the fifth century B.C. and the second century A.D. that presents a spiritual gospel of values, ethics, devotion, and principles of self-development toward the goal of enlightenment and liberation (*moksha*).

Bhakti Yoga: The Yoga of devotion.

Bhasma: Ayurvedic medicinal incinerated mineral, metal ash, or oxide.

Bhastrika: A therapeutic form of intense breathing resembling the action of a bellows.

Bhava: Becoming.

Bhavana: The process, sometimes using a mortar and pestle, used to enhance or improve the qualities of a substance; meditation; techniques of self-development.

Bhavaprakasha: 16th century Ayurvedic text delineating a range of medical treatments.

Bheda: The stage of pathogenesis that is the differentiation stage.

Bhishak: Ayurvedic physician.

Bhrajaka Pitta: The subdosha of *Pitta* giving color and warmth to the skin.

Bhujanasana: The Yoga posture (cobralike) beneficial for *Tarpaka Kapha.*

Bhuta: One of the five great gross Elements that compose all physical matter: Ether, Air, Fire, Water, and Earth.

Bhutagni: The digestive fire residing in the liver that processes the Elements, especially for the nutrition of the sensory organs.

Bibhitake: Medicinal fruit (*Terminalia belerica).*

Bhutavidya: Psychiatry, one of the eight branches of Ayurveda.

Black Pepper: Spice (*Piper nigrum).*

Bodhaka Kapha: The subdosha of *Kapha* associated with taste and contained in saliva.

Brahma: The first god of the Hindu trinity; god as creator of the universe.

Brahmacharya: The appropriate control and regulation of sexual energy and functioning.

Brahman: God as Absolute transcendence.

Brahmanas: Texts of the ancient Vedas that are chiefly concerned with details of the ritual sacrifices performed by the ancient Brahmins.

Brahmanda: The macrocosm; the manifest universe.

Brahmin: A Hindu priest; a member of the first caste of Vedic society, the Brahmin class consisting of priests, scholars, philosophers, and spiritual devotees.

Brhadaranyaka: The earliest known Upanishad describing Yoga practice and meditation.

Brihat: Enormous, vast.

Brimhana: Toning, strengthening, and supplementation therapy; one of the two broad classes of Ayurvedic therapies; see LANGHANA.

Buddhi: The faculty of intelligent discrimination emanating from pure consciousness that is potentially accessible to all individuals to enhance cognition and, therefore, widen the range of available consciousness.

Cardamom: Spice (*Elettaria cardamomum*).

Castor oil: Medicinal oil (*Ricinus communis*).

Catabolism: The metabolic breakdown of cellular and tissue substance.

Cayenne: Red pepper (*Capsicum spp*).

Chakra: A subtle energy center located along the spinal canal and brain (*sushumna*); *Prana* and *Kundalini* are concentrated here; major nodes at which spirit interpenetrates with matter in the body.

Chakshu: Eyes.

Chala: Agitated, mobile.

Charaka: One of the most famous of Ayurvedic physicians (c. seventh century B.C.) and author of foundational text by the same name.

Charaka Samhita: The textbook of Ayurvedic medicine compiled by the school of Charaka in the first millennium B.C.

Chela: Student, pupil, or spiritual disciple.

Chi: The life force; *Prana;* also *Qi.*

Chikitsa: Therapy, treatment.

Chit: Absolute consciousness.

Chitta: The aspect of mind that regulates perception, thinking, and memory and is virtually identical to *Manas*.

Chitam: A technical term denoting the range of differing levels of consciousness, i.e., unconscious, conventionally conscious or alert, and superconscious.

Chyvanprash: Herbomineral jam with tonifying and rejuvenating properties.

Cinnamon: Spice (*Cinnamomum zeylanicum*).

Coriander: Spice (*Coriandrum sativum*).

Cumin: Spice (*Cuminum cyminum*).

Daiva: Spiritual.

Daiva Chikitsa: Spiritual therapy.

Dandelion: Food and herb (*Taraxacum officinale*).

Danta: Teeth.

Darshana: Vision, viewpoint, philosophy, ideological system, and worldview.

Deha: The physical body that is well nourished.

Deha prakruti: The constitution or body type developed and stabilized at maturity.

Devi: Deity companion of Shiva; also known as *Shakti*.

Dhanvantari: Vedic deity, regarded as the father of Ayurveda.

Dhara kala: The membrane specific to each of the seven bodily tissues that has nutritive, metabolic, protective, and structural functions.

Dharana: Focused concentration; stabilization.

Dharma: The lawful order within the universe; one's values, ethics, morals, destiny, fate, duty, or obligations.

Dhatu: The substantive root or source of a tissue; the tissue, itself; the physical body is composed of seven *dhatus* or tissues: (1) *rasa* (plasma); (2) *rakta* (blood); (3) *mamsa* (muscle); (4) *asthi* (bone); (5) *meda* (fat); (6) *majja* (nerve-marrow); and (7) *shukra* (reproductive).

Dhatuagni: The metabolic or digestive fire that processes tissue elements.

Dhatu kshaya: Tissue loss.

Dhauti: Yoga procedure to cleanse the stomach.

Dhi: Wisdom.

Dhooma: Therapeutic smoking of herbal preparations.

Dhruti: Patience, impulse control, and will power.

Dhuta: Shaking off and becoming free of bondage to desire and to the inordinate attachment to material possessions.

Dhyana: Meditation.

Dinacharya: The daily routine of personal hygiene.

Dipana: Techniques and herbs used to stimulate the digestive fire, the *Agni*.

Doosha: Vitiated and damaged tissues, organs, or channels; also spelled *dusha* and *dushya*.

Dosha: A fundamental bioenergetic principle and substance that regulates homeostasis in biological organisms; *doshas*, by nature, are dynamic and protective, and constantly become vitiated or stressed; there are three *doshas*: (1) *Vata*; (2) *Pitta*; and (3) *Kapha*.

Doshavidha Pariksha: The clinical examination of a patient using 10 parameters.
Drava: Liquid.
Dravya: Substance.
Dravyaguna Shastra: Indian Materia Medica, pharmacognosy, and pharmacology; Ayurvedic medicine.
Dridhikarana: Hardening.
Duhkha: Suffering and pain.
Dushika: Sclerotic fluid of the eyes.
Dushya: Tissues, organs, and channels affected by vitiated *doshas;* also spelled *dusha;* see DOOSHA.
Dvesha: Repulsion; aversion for unpleasant things.
Ekagra: The state of mind that is singularly focused.
Emmenagogue: Medicinal substance that promotes blood circulation.
Fennel: Spice (*Foeniculum vulgans).*
Flaxseed: Medicinal oil (*Linum usitatissimum).*
Ganesha: The divine son of Shiva; the deity of wisdom and the remover of obstacles.
Garbhashaya: Womb.
Gati: The particular quality of a movement.
Ghandha: Smell, aroma.
Ghee: Clarified butter.
Ginger: Medicinal herbal root (*Zingiber officinale).*
Gorasa: Dairy products.
Gotu Kola: Herb (*Hydrocotyle asiatica).*
Grahana: Nose.
Grahani: The small intestine.
Guduchi: Herb (*Tinospora cordifolia).*
Guggulu: Resin (*Commiphora mukul).*
Guna: Attribute or quality; adjectival description of the physical and chemical properties of a substance; all material substances can be characterized by *gunas* or attributes and qualities; 10 pairs are described: (1) cold / hot; (2) wet / dry; (3) heavy / light; (4) gross / subtle; (5) dense / liquid; (6) stable / mobile; (7) dull / sharp; (8) soft / hard; (9) smooth / rough; (10) cloudy / clear; also referred to as *gurvadi gunas.*
Guru: Heavy; teacher, guide.

Gurvadi gunas: The attributes and qualities that are associated with material substances; see GUNA.

Halasana: The Yogic plow posture.

Hamsagati: Pulse movements that are swanlike that are characteristic of *Kapha*.

Haritaki: Medicinal fruit (*Terminalia chebula)*.

Harita varga: Raw vegetables.

Hatha Yoga: The Yoga of physical postures (*asanas)* and breath control (*pranayama*).

Hetu: Cause.

Hima: Cold.

Homa: Sacrificial offering put into a ritual fire; also *yajna*.

Humor: An older term denoting the concept of *dosha,* a primary bioenergetic regulatory principle and substance in the body.

Hridaya: Heart; the connotation of heart as a center of power.

Iccha: Desire.

Iksuvikara: Sugars.

Indriyas: The five sense organs (ears, skin, eyes, tongue, and nose) and the five motor organs of action (mouth, hands, feet, penis, and anus).

Ishvara: The manifestation of God or the Absolute having personal characteristics.

Jala: Water.

Jalauka: Therapeutic bloodletting using medically supervised applications of leeches.

Janma prakruti: The constitutional conformation present at birth.

Japa: Repetition.

Jatamansi: Herb (*Nardostachys spp)*.

Jatharagni: The primary digestive fire centered in the stomach and small intestine.

Jihva: Tongue.

Jing: A fundamental principle in Chinese medicine connoting the primary essence of the body, the fundamental substance of organic life that underlies all vital development.

Jiva: The spirit or soul as the embodied individual self that identifies with the body and the mind.

Jnana Yoga: The Yoga of knowledge.

Jnanendriya: The five sensory organs of perception: ears, skin, eyes, mouth / tongue, and nose.

Jyotish: Vedic Astrology.

Kaivalya: Liberation from material existence as the ultimate *samadhi* of Yoga practice.

Kala: Time; sometimes used as a synonym for death.

Kala Parinama: The effects that the passage of time (age, aging, seasons, etc.) produces in the natural world.

Kale Kapota: The "land and pigeon" theory that explains the process of bodily tissue formation.

Kali: Black; the fierce and ominous appearing female deity; the companion of Shiva who, like him, acts as a destroyer, often with positive connotations, i.e., destroyer of ignorance.

Kama: Sensual desire or pleasure; in the *Rig-Veda*, the first impulse that initiated primal creation.

Kampa: Tremor.

Kandara: Fascia; tendons.

Kapha: The bioenergetic Water *dosha*; one of the body's three fundamental regulatory principles whose main function is that of providing cohesion, binding, and containment.

Kara: Rough.

Karana: Entirely spiritual; pre-energetic, causal, seed, magnetic, or soul dimension of created reality.

Karma: Mental or physical action and / or its consequences.

Karma Yoga: The Yoga of action and service.

Karmendriya: The five motor organs of action: mouth / speech, hands, feet, genitals, and anus.

Karuna: Compassion.

Kashaya: The astringent taste; the residue left in consciousness by sensual pleasure; also spelled *kasaya*.

Katha Upanishad: An early Upanishad that is believed to be the first formal text to use the term *Yoga*.

Kathina: Hard.

Katu: The pungent or spicy taste.

Kaumarabhritya: The Obstetric, Gynecologic, and Pediatric branch of Ayurveda.

Kaya: The physical body that actively transforms and assimilates nutrition.

Kayachikitsa: Internal Medicine, one of the eight branches of Ayurveda.

Kaya Kalpa: Rejuvenation of the body; a specialty treatment within Ayurveda.

Kedara Kula: The channel irrigation theory that explains the mechanisms of bodily tissue formation.

Kensho: The Zen Buddhist understanding of self-realization and enlightenment as a gradually evolving process.

Kervaigunya: A weak or pathological area in a tissue or channel that may become the ground for disease.

Kesha: Hair.

Khamalas: Wastes produced as byproducts of muscle tissue formation.

Khara: Rough.

Khust: Dietary restrictions.

Kitchari: Wholesome, balance, and cleansing meal specifically consisting of Basmati rice, yellow split mung lentils, vegetables, and light spices.

Kleda: Nonspecific, subtle waste products that result from the formation of the seven primary bodily tissues (*dhatus*).

Kledaka Kapha: The subdosha of *Kapha* that aids digestion in the stomach.

Kledana: Moistening.

Kopana: That which aggravates a *dosha*.

Kosha: Sheath or covering; one of the five sheaths comprising the individual and having *atman* at its core.

Koshta: Hollow spaces in the body, particularly the central gastrointestinal tract.

Koshta Marga: The gastrointestinal tract.

Krimi: Germs, bacteria, viruses, fungi, parasites, and other infectious organisms.

Kritana: Cooked food preparations.

Kshalana: Cleansing action.

Kshatriya: The second caste of Vedic society composed of warriors, politicians, nobility, and royalty.

Ksheera Dadhi: The direct, transformative sequence theory that explains the formation of bodily tissues.

Ksheta: Field; womb.

Kundalini: Spiritual energy, related to the power of consciousness, figuratively depicted as the serpent power sleeping at the base of the spine available to travel upward through the *sushumna* and energize the *chakras* thereby further awakening consciousness.

Kushala: The Buddhist notion of wholesomeness that includes aspects of working through and dissolving one's *karma.*

Laghu: Light.

Lakshmi: The Deity of fortune and companion of Vishnu.

Langhana: Reduction therapy; one of the two broad classes of Ayurvedic treatments; see BRIMHANA.

Laya Yoga: The Yoga of intense veneration using the vehicle of meditatively activating the *Kundalini* energies to bring about dissolution and merging with the Absolute.

Lavana: The salty taste.

Lekhana: Scraping action.

Lepana: Adhering and binding action.

Licorice: Herbal root (*Glycyrrhiza glabra).*

Madhava Nidana: Ayurvedic text (c. A.D. 700–1100) delineating the diagnosis of disease types.

Madhya: Adulthood from adolescence through middle age.

Madhyama Marga: The middle pathway within the body through which diseases travel as they penetrate into the deeper tissues and vital organs.

Madhura: The sweet taste.

Madhuvinashini: Herb (*Gymnema sylvestre).*

Madya: Wines and spirits.

Mahabhutanis: The five great gross Elements; also spelled *mahabhuta*(*s*); see BHUTA.

Maha gunas: Sattva, Rajas, and *Tamas;* these are the three fundamental, highly rarefied potentials within *Prakriti* (manifest nature) whose magnitude in any substance determines its specific nature, tendencies, and actions; some combination of *Maha gunas* are present in all dimensions of human life ranging from the biological through the psychological to the spiritual.

Maha Srotas: The gastrointestinal tract.

Mahat: The first and enduring manifestation of cosmic intelligence in the universe.

Mahayana Buddhism: The branch of Buddhism, arising in the first century A.D., that emphasizes the attainment of enlightenment for the sake of the welfare of all beings; developing wisdom (*prajna*) and compassion (*karuna*) through ethical behavior constitute fundamental values.

Majja: Bone marrow and nerve tissue.

Majjadhara kala: The membranes of the nervous system.

Majjavaha Srotas: The nervous system.

Mala: Waste material of the body; also *malas;* Hindu prayer beads.

Mamsa: Muscle tissue.

Mamsadhara kala: The membranes of the muscles.

Mamsavaha Srotas: The channels of circulation of the muscles.

Manas: That aspect of the inner cognitive organ (*antakarana*) roughly equated with mind as the faculty of the thinking apparatus; the conditioned, sensate, and thinking mind; mentation; mind as an organ of desire.

Manasa: Relating to the mind; psychological; bodily illness due to psychological causes.

Manda: Slow, dull; rice water.

Manipura Chakra: The energy node located in the region of the navel.

Mandagni: The pathologically lowered state of the digestive fire or *Agni.*

Mandukagati: Pulse movements with froglike qualities that are characteristic of *Pitta.*

Manomaya Kosha: The mental and emotional sheath; the third of five layers or sheaths that composes the individual human being.

Manovaha Srotas: The channels of circulation associated with mental processes.

Mantra: Originally, a sacred sound or word used to enhance meditation; a power-laden syllable or series of syllables used to imbue an action with auspicious transformative qualities.

Mantra Yoga: The Yoga that uses *japa* or repetition of a mantra as a primary self-development technique.

Mara: Passion, desire, murder, destruction.

Marana: A passing away or qualitative change such as death; an Ayurvedic mineral preparation.
Marga: A specific pathway or tract.
Marma: A vital, energetic area located on the surface of the body.
Marut: Another name for *Vayu* or the Air Element; the name of the Vedic storm god.
Maruta-sevana: Therapeutic windbathing.
Maya: The conventional and erroneous experience of believing that first impressions or appearances constitute the entire nature of a thing; i.e., the mind's subjective deception or illusory beliefs, especially when cognition fails to recognize that consciousness is at the base of reality and that unity rather than diversity pervades the universe.
Medas: The fat tissue; also spelled *Meda.*
Medodhara kala: The membranes around fat tissue.
Medovaha Srotas: The channels of circulation of adipose tissue.
Misra: Ancient Vedic name for present-day Egypt.
Moksha: The state of liberation from bondage to worldly attachments and to the experience of desire; freedom from *karma* and *samsara;* the highest goal of life.
Mrudu: Soft.
Muladhara Chakra: The base or foundational energy node located between the root of the genitals and the anus.
Mutra: Urine.
Mutravaha Srotas: The urinary system.
Nadi: Channel, tube, vessel, canal; Ayurvedic term for the pulse.
Nadi Pariksha: Ayurvedic technique of examining the pulse.
Nakha: Nails.
Nanatmaja: A disease state characterized by the involvement of one vitiated *dosha.*
Nastika darshana: Any worldview that does not recognize the Vedas as lawful and authoritative; observant Hindus consider such viewpoints as unorthodox.
Nasya: Administration of medicinals via the nasal canal.
Neem: Herb (*Azadirachta indica).*
Nidana: Etiology; cause; link; and diagnosis.
Nija: Endogenous causes of disease.
Nirguna: Without attributes or qualities.
Nirama: The state of *doshas* that are free of *Ama.*

Niruha Basti: Ayurvedic enema therapy primarily containing herbal water decoctions.

Nirvana: In many Eastern *darshanas* or worldviews, the highest goal to be achieved by an individual, especially by using spiritual practices, i.e., meditation; degrees of extinction of bondage to the impermanent and transitory; recognition of one's pure identity or oneness with the Absolute.

Niyama: In Yoga, correct or right actions and personal observances.

Nutmeg: Spice (*Myristica fragrans)*.

Nyaya: One of the six orthodox Hindu philosophical systems that uses reason, logic, and analytic thinking to pursue knowledge.

Ojas: The bioenergetic bodily material that contains the life force (*Prana*) and serves the vital functions that maintain the body's energy reserve and proper immune status.

Oshadhi: Plant; herb; also *aushadhi.*

Pachaka Pitta: The subdosha of *Pitta* or the *Agni* that resides in the stomach and small intestine and helps regulate primary digestion.

Pad: Feet.

Padmasana: Yoga posture; the lotus pose.

Pali: An Indian dialect derived from Sanskrit in which the canonical Buddhist texts, especially those of *Theravada* Buddhism, are composed.

Pancha: Five.

Panchakarma: The five primary cleansing actions of Ayurvedic purification therapy: *vamana, virechana, basti, nasya,* and *rakta moksha.*

Pancha Mahabhutani: The five great gross Elements: Ether, Air, Fire, Water, and Earth.

Pancha Tanmatras: The five subtle essences energizing the five great gross Elements.

Pancha Tattvas: The causal, soul, seed, magnetic, and most spiritual level of the origin of the five great gross Elements and the sensory organs.

Pachana: Techniques and herbs that digest and reduce *Ama* and toxins.

Pani: Hands.

Parada: Mercury.

Paramartha-satya: Ultimate and absolute truth; the realization of the unity underlying the apparent diversity that characterizes the ordinary experience of the phenomenal world.

Pariksha: Examination; diagnosis.

Paschatakarma: The final techniques used after formal *Panchakarma* is completed.

Patanjali: The codifier of one of the six major orthodox Hindu philosophical systems, classical Yoga (c. second century B.C.-second century A.D.).

Pathya: Proper and wholesome diet and lifestyle.

Payu: Anus.

Peppermint: Herb (*Mentha piperita).*

Peya: Thin rice soup.

Phala: Fruit.

Picchila: Cloudy, sticky, and slimy.

Pinda: The microcosm; the individual.

Pippali: Herb (*Piper longum).*

Pitta: The bioenergetic Fire *dosha;* one of the body's three fundamental regulatory principles whose main function is that of transformation, penetrating heat production, and digestion.

Prabha: Bodily luster.

Prabhava: The special action of an herb that goes beyond the expectable effects of its taste, attributes, and actions.

Prachhana: Therapeutic blood letting using sharp instruments.

Prajna: The innate wisdom that emanates from pure consciousness.

Prajna-aparadha: The natural and intrinsic tendency for human consciousness and wisdom to be in error especially when the underlying unity of reality is forgotten; the influence of *Manas* (ordinary mental processes) on overall cognition.

Prakopa: The aggravated and excited state of a vitiated *dosha.*

Prakriti: Primordial Nature or Matter that is initially undifferentiated but then gradually organizes to become energetic and manifest as a multiplicity of substances composed of energy and matter.

Prakruti: The individual body type or constitution of a person; the structural and functional expression of the individual's genetic code.

Prakruti Pariksha: The process of evaluating the specific *prakruti* of an individual.

Prakupita: The action of vitiated *Vata* that pathologically propels *Ama* and toxins into the body's deep tissue structures.

Pramana: Any reliable and trustworthy technique for ascertaining knowledge.

Prana: The life force, *chi;* the life force along with its vehicle, the breath; the subdosha and main form of *Vata* associated with inhalation.

Pranamaya Kosha: The breath sheath containing *Prana;* the second of five layers or sheaths that compose the individual human being.

Pranavaha Srotas: The respiratory system; the channels of circulation of *Prana.*

Pranayama: The technique of regulating the breathing process; a primary phase of Yoga exercise.

Prapaka: Primary digestion; also *avasthapaka.*

Prapatti: Surrender to spiritual life.

Prasad: Food that is blessed, purified, and used in ritual offerings; grace or blessing received.

Prasadana: Solidifying and becoming dense.

Prasanna: Satisfied.

Prasara: Spreading.

Prash: Ayurvedic herbal jam or jelly.

Prashama: Alleviation or pacification of previously excited *doshas.*

Prashna: Contemplative exercises in the form of questions pondering the meaning of life and the nature of reality.

Pratiloma: The abnormal direction of flow within a channel of circulation.

Pratimarshya: The intranasal administration of small amounts of therapeutic oil.

Pratyahara: The practice of attempting to withdraw the attention that emanates from the senses away from objects in the external world in order to discipline the mind; an advanced stage in Yoga.

Pratyaksha: The direct sensory perception, using the five senses, of objects in the external world; evidence from the senses.

Prerana: Stimulating.

Prinana: A function of the plasma tissue that results in a sense of satisfaction and well-being following proper nutrition.

Prithvi: The Earth Element.

Purana: Contentment, filling.

Puranas: The body of Puranic literature; ancient, devotional stories referring to legends concerning the gods, Brahma, Vishnu, and Shiva, but including some royal genealogies, dating from about A.D. 320–520 through the Middle Ages.

Purgation: Strong laxative action; one of the Ayurvedic *Panchakarma* treatments; *virechana.*

Purisha: The bodily waste product of feces.

Purishadhara kala: The special membranes of the colon.

Purishavaha Srotas: The fecal elimination system.

Purusha: In the orthodox *Sankhya* worldview, absolute and unlimited consciousness and pure spirit characterized as completely immaterial and unmanifest.

Purushartha: According to the Vedas, the four prime goals toward which each individual has the opportunity to strive: *dharma, artha, kama,* and *moksha.*

Purva: Preceding; premonitory; prodromal.

Purvakarma: The preparatory techniques used before formal *Panchakarma* is begun.

Purva Mimamsa: One of the six orthodox Hindu *darshanas* or worldviews that emphasizes the meaningfulness of the words of the Vedic scriptures and their prescribed ritual obligations.

Purva Rupa: Prodromal signs and symptoms of a disease.

Qi: The life force; *Prana;* also *chi.*

Raga: The qualities of passion that evoke a sense of attraction.

Raja: Royal or best; menstrual fluid.

Rajas: One of the three *Maha gunas;* the highly rarefied principle of energetic transformation, transmutation, and turbulence.

Rajasic: Having the attribute of *Rajas.*

Rakta: The blood tissue.

Raktadhara kala: The special membranes of the circulatory system; includes endothelial lining of blood vessels.

Raktavaha Srotas: The blood circulatory system.

Rakta Moksha: Therapeutic blood letting; therapeutic blood purification; one of the Ayurvedic *Panchakarma* procedures.

Ranjaka Pitta: The subdosha of *Pitta* associated with erythrocyte formation and transformations within the liver.

Rasa: Plasma; taste of a substance perceived by the tongue; essence; spiritual enjoyment.

Rasavaha Srotas: The channels of circulation of the *rasa.*

Rasayana: Antiaging and rejuvenation, one of the eight branches of Ayurveda; also a rejuvenative herbomineral preparation.

Rasayana Chikitsa: Rejuvenation treatment.

Rig-Veda: The preeminent and most ancient compilation of the four primary Vedas of the Hindus from which Ayurveda is derived in part; its origins are prehistoric; it contains 1,028 hymns that are the basis for all orthodox Hindu worldviews.

Rig: Hymn; also spelled *rik.*

Rishi: An inspired seer; originally, one of many to whom the ancient Vedas were revealed.

Ritam: The innate law and order of the universe.

Ritu: Season.

Ritucharya: Lifestyle regimen adjusted according to the specific season in order to maintain proper doshic balance.

Roga: Disease.

Roga Pariksha: The examination of disease.

Ropana: Healing action.

Rupa: Symptom; sight.

Ruksha: Dry.

Rukshana: Therapeutic drying therapies that reduce bodily fluids and tissue substance.

Sabda: Sound; hearing; teaching, scholarly testimony; also spelled *shabda.*

Sadhaka Pitta: The subdosha of *Pitta* located in the heart and the brain.

Sadhana: Spiritual practices used as a means to achieve self-development.

Sadvritta: Ethical regimens that guide daily living.

Saguna: Having attributes and qualities (*gunas*).

Sahasrara Chakra: The crown energy node located above the top of the head.

Saka: Vegetables.

Sama: The state of the *doshas* when contaminated with *Ama.*

Sama Agni: The digestive fire or *Agni* in its balanced and optimal state.

Samadhi: The refined state of consciousness marked by degrees of freedom from illusion, error, and dualistic experience.

Saman: Songs and melodies; especially those found in the Vedas (*Sama-Veda*), used to transmit the hymns of the *Rig-Veda*.

Samana Vata: The subdosha of *Vata* associated with peristalsis and digestion in the gastrointestinal tract.

Samanya: Like increases like; one of two basic principles of Ayurvedic treatment; universal applicability; general; see also VISHESHA.

Samanyaja: A disease state characterized by the involvement of two vitiated *doshas*.

Sama-Veda: One of the four primary Vedas consisting of 1,549 songs or verses that accompanied the preparation and offering of ritual sacrifices.

Samhanana: Bodily conformation and structural integrity.

Samhita: A unified collection; usually a collection of sacred, philosophical, or medical teachings.

Samidhanya: Legumes, beans, and lentils.

Samkalpa: Conception, will, motivation, intention, synthesis.

Sammurchanna: The pathological amalgamation of *Ama* and *dushya*.

Sampropti: Pathogenesis; the stages of the disease process.

Samsara: Cycles of repetition; pulsed cyclic rebirth; the impermanent phenomenal world.

Samsarga: A disease state characterized by the involvement of two vitiated *doshas*.

Samskara: Conditioning; the impressions, changes, and layers of modification produced by thoughts and action.

Samsarjana Krama: A specific, graduated dietary intake used after formal *Panchakarma* is completed.

Samvarana: Gross or dense covering.

Samvritti-satya: Conventional and relative truth ascertained by ordinary, discursive but nonreflective mentation.

Samyama: Self-discipline through rigorous physical and mental constraint.

Sanchaya: Accumulation or buildup of *doshas* in the initial stages of the disease process.

Sandhis: Bony joints.

Sandra: Dense; congealing.

Sankhya: One of the six major orthodox systems of Hindu philosophy that enumerates details of the process of cosmic evolution.

Sannikrustha: Agents that cause the instantaneous manifestation of a disease.

Sannipata: A disease state characterized by involvement of three vitiated *doshas.*

Sara: Optimal quality.

Sarangadhara Samhita: 14th century text presenting the Ayurvedic technique of pulse diagnosis.

Sarasvati: The companion of *Brahma*; the deity associated with the development of speech, scholarship, music, and the arts.

Sarpagati: Snakelike pulse movements characteristic of *Vata.*

Sat: Absolute, eternal, and unchanging being.

Satsanga: Associating with those that are wholesome.

Sattva: One of the three *Maha gunas*; the highly rarefied principle of consciousness, intelligence, harmony, equilibrium, optimal balance, clarity, purity, and lightness.

Sattvic: Having the quality of *Sattva.*

Satya: Truth.

Satyam: Truth.

Satya Buddhi: The ascertainment of truth; the state of *samadhi.*

Satyma: Wholesome.

Saumya: The cool, cold, and wet seasons; in the United States, usually fall and winter; see also VISARGA.

Sesame: Nutritive and medicinal oil (*Sesamum indicum).*

Shakha: The limbs or extremities; the peripheral compact tissues.

Shakha Marga: The bodily pathway within which disease travels to reach the compact tissues, especially those of the four limbs.

Shakti: Power, force, energy; the companion (*Devi*) of Shiva.

Shalakya Tantra: Otolaryngology and Ophthalmology, branches of Ayurveda.

Shalyatantra: Surgery, one of the eight branches of Ayurveda.

Samavaya: Unified interplay of component parts.

Shamana: Therapeutic techniques that reduce toxic *Ama* and excess vitiated *doshas.*
Sharira: Physical body that experiences wear and tear.
Shastra: Treatise or textbook consisting of ideas, beliefs, theories, rituals, or scientific formulations.
Shatavari: Herb (*Asparagus racemosus).*
Shirobasti: Therapeutic oil retention on the top of the head.
Shirodhara: Therapeutic oil drip to the forehead.
Shita: Cool.
Shiva: One of the triune deities in Hinduism; the deity of dissolution and transformation, i.e., impurity into purity, ignorance into understanding.
Shlakshna: Smooth.
Shlathana: Softening and loosening.
Shleshaka Kapha: The subdosha of *Kapha* composed of joint and synovial fluids; also SLESHAKA KAPHA.
Shlesma: Ancient name for *Kapha.*
Shlesmadhara kala: The special membrane associated with the plasma; also spelled *sleshakadhara kala.*
Shodhana: Ayurvedic purification therapy.
Shoshana: Absorption.
Shrotra: Ears.
Shuddha: Purity, unadulterated; a principal feature of *Sattva;* also spelled *shuddhi, suddhi.*
Shuddhi Kriya: The purification techniques unique to Yoga practice.
Shudra: One of the Vedic social classes composed of skilled and unskilled laborers.
Shukra: Reproductive fluids; semen.
Shukra Beej: Paternal seed or genetic material.
Shukradhara kala: The special membrane of the reproductive system.
Shukravaha Srotas: The male reproductive system.
Siddhi: Success; exceptional abilities or powers that may appear as byproducts of spiritual practices.
Sira: Blood vessels.
Siravyadha: Therapeutic blood letting using sterile syringes.
Sleshakadhara kala: *Shlesmadhara kala.*

Sleshaka Kapha: The subdosha of *Kapha* composed of joint and synovial fluids.

Smriti: Memory or recollection associated with knowledge derived from tradition; the bulk of commentaries on the primary Vedas; also spelled *smruti.*

Snayus: Ligaments.

Snehana: Therapeutic procedures using oils and fats as in massage or therapeutic ingestion.

Snigdhda: Oily.

Soma: In the *Rig-Veda,* a sacred plant and its juice used by the Brahmins for ritual purposes; the exact nature of *Soma,* in current times, is ambiguous.

Spandana Sankhya: Pulse rate.

Sparsha: Touch.

Sparshana: Contact by touch; examination by palpation.

Srotas: The channels of circulation through which the seven bodily tissue elements (*dhatus*) dynamically move.

Srotorhodha: Obstruction of the channels of circulation.

Sruti: The revealed sacred Vedic scriptures originally "heard" by the *rishis;* the orthodox Vedas; also spelled *shruti.*

Stambhana: Cooling.

Sthana Samshraya: The pathological deposition of *Ama* into vitiated tissue.

Stanya: Breast milk; also spelled *sthanya.*

Stanyavaha Srotas: The channels of circulation of the female lactation system.

Sthira: Stable.

Sthula: Gross; coarse; physical; and material.

Sthula sharira: The physical body.

Suka Dhanya: Cereals and grains.

Sukha: Happiness.

Sukha Sadhya: Disease that has a favorable prognosis.

Sukshma: Subtle; energetic.

Sushruta: Ancient Ayurvedic surgeon (c. seventh century B.C.) who composed the standard Ayurvedic text, *Sushruta Samhita.*

Sushruta Samhita: The classic Ayurvedic textbook written by *Sushruta* that highlights the significance of the blood and the importance of surgical in additional to other medical techniques.

Sushumna: The primary and central energy channel running along the spine and brain that contains the *Kundalini* and along which the seven *chakras* are located.

Susukshma: Having the highest degree of immateriality or subtlety within created nature.

Surya Namaskara: The "sun salutation" yogic exercise; also *suryasana*.

Sutra: A terse aphorism that summarizes sacred knowledge.

Svadhisthana Chakra: The energy node at the root of the genital region.

Svadhyaya: The study of sacred scripture.

Swastha: Health and well-being.

Swasthavritta: Ayurvedic lifestyle regimens for promoting optimal health.

Sweda: Sweat.

Swedana: Ayurvedic procedure to promote therapeutic sweating; also referred to as sudation therapy.

Swedanavaha Srotas: Channels of circulation that carry sweat.

Tail: Medicated oil.

Tamas: One of the three *Maha gunas;* the highly rarefied principle that engenders inertia, density, and dulling.

Tamasic: Having the quality of *Tamas.*

Tanmatra: One of the five subtle or energetic states that act as precursor to the formation of the five great gross Elements, especially as they contribute to the formation of the five senses.

Tantra: Technique, method, mechanism; a development in Hinduism specifically concerned with the transformative power of *Kundalini* energy; the dialogues between Shiva and his companion, Shakti or Devi; Charaka uses this term in describing the structure of Ayurveda as compiled in his text.

Tapas: Rigorous spiritual cultivation that involves self-discipline, austerity, mortification, and internally heat-generating impulses.

Tarpaka Kapha: The subdosha of *Kapha* located in the cerebrospinal fluids.

Tarpana: Observances and exercise that address recognition of one's ancestral heritage in an attempt to disengage from bondage to a predetermined legacy.

Tattva: A fundamental principle or truth within a *darshana* or worldview.

Tejas: The subtle energetic form of *Pitta;* the Fire Element.

Theravada Buddhism: The branch of Buddhism, arising between the sixth and first century B.C., that emphasizes individual self-development through ascetic renunciation as a means to liberation (*moksha*) from desire and the transitory attachments of the material world.

Tikta: The bitter taste.

Tikshna: Penetrating; sharp.

Tikshna Agni: The pathologically high state of the digestive fire or *Agni.*

Tridosha: The three *doshas: Vata, Pitta,* and *Kapha* (VPK).

Triguna: The three *Maha gunas*: *Sattva, Rajas,* and *Tamas.*

Triphala: Famous Ayurvedic triple herbal combination: *Haritaki, Amalaki,* and *Bibhitaki.*

Tripti: Contentment, satiation.

Trishna: Desire and craving.

Trit: Fluid restriction.

Tulsi: Indian holy basil (*Ocimum sanctum).*

Turmeric: Spice (*Curcuma longa).*

Tvak: Skin.

Udaka: Water.

Udakavaha Srotas: The channels of circulation that carry water.

Udana Vata: The subdosha of *Vata* associated with expiration.

Umada: Mental disorders.

Upadana: Attachment, desire, and the formation of bonds to material and worldly experience.

Upadhatu: The secondary or accessory tissue elements that result from the formation of the seven primary bodily tissues (*dhatus*).

Upadrava: Complications of a disease.

Upamana: Analogy.

Upanishads: Ancient Hindu scriptures that are termed *Vedanta* or the later parts of the Vedas.

Upashaya: Relief of symptoms after a suitably appropriate treatment intervention.

Upashta: Genitalia.

Upayoga samstha: Dietary and nutritional guidelines.

Upaveda: One of the subsidiary, subsequent, or secondary Vedas, i.e., Ayurveda, an accessory to the *Athara-Veda.*

Upchaya: Physical build; suitability.

Up-pa-sad: Sanskrit term describing the seating of a pupil across from a teacher when engaged in the study of ancient scripture.

Ushna: Hot.

Utkleshana: Liquefied vitiated *doshas* that are ready to be eliminated via *Panchakarma.*

Utpadaka: Vitiation, impairment, and disturbance, especially of a *dosha.*

Utsaha: Endurance, vitality.

Uttarakarma: Procedures used after formal *Panchakarma* is completed.

Uttara Mimansa: *Advaita Vedanta.*

Vac: Speech; see VAK.

Vaidya: Physician.

Vagbhata: Ayurvedic physician who wrote major medical text *Ashtanga Hridaya* (c. 700–500 A.D.).

Vaishya: The Vedic social class of merchants and agriculturists that provided materials and goods within that society.

Vajikarana: Reproductive and aphrodisiac medicine, one of the eight branches of Ayurveda; also an aphrodisiac substance or substance that contributes to enhancing one's capacity to produce progeny.

Vaisheshika: One of the oldest of the six major orthodox Hindu worldviews that attempts to delineate a scientific categorization of nature.

Vak: Mouth, speech, voice, language; goddess of words in the Vedas; also spelled *vac, vach.*

Vamana: One of the five *Panchakarma* purification treatments that involve therapeutic emesis.

Varna: Complexion, color with symbolic meaning.

Vasa: Muscle fat.

Vata: The bioenergetic *dosha* of Air; one of the body's three fundamental regulatory principles whose main function is that of propulsion and movement.

Vaya: Age.

Vayas: Lifespan.

Vayayama Shakti: Energy level.

Vayu: In the Vedas, the deity of air; the Air Element; synonymous with *Vata dosha.*

Vedas: The knowledge, wisdom, and sacred teachings revealed to the ancient seers. The primary Vedas comprise the four main Vedic texts: *Rig-Veda, Sama-Veda, Yajur-Veda,* and *Athara-Veda.*

Vedanga: Limbs of the Vedas; supplementary texts to the ancient Vedas.

Vedanta: The end of the Vedas; found in texts such as the *Upanishads.*

Vega-dharana: Natural, physiological urges.

Vidahi: Overly stimulating.

Vihara: Lifestyle practices.

Vijnana: Pure intelligence; proper consciousness of reality in everyday living.

Vijnanomaya Kosha: The intelligence-wisdom sheath; the fourth of five layers or sheaths that compose the individual human being.

Vikalpa: Unruly; disordered; false imagination; the attributes of a *dosha* that are abnormally increased in disease.

Vikara: Diversification; the differing manifestations that develop as a disease progresses.

Vikruti: The current, imbalanced state of one's *prakruti* or constitution that results from doshic imbalances and the accumulation of toxicity in the body.

Vikruti Pariksha: The examination of the imbalanced constitution.

Vilepi: Thick rice soup.

Vilodana: Liquefying and dissolving.

Vimarga gamana: The pathological flow of bodily substances outside of their proper channels of circulation.

Vipaka: The postdigestive effect of an ingested substance after assimilation.

Viparita-Bhavana: The ordinary and erroneous belief that the visible world of appearances constitutes the whole of reality; a function of *Manas*.

Viprakrustha: Agents that produce disease after a long incubation period.

Virechana: Ayurvedic purgation therapy as one aspect of *Panchakarma* purification.

Virya: The energetic power of a substance characterized on a spectrum ranging from hot to cold.

Visada: Clear.

Visarga Kala: The wet seasons; generally fall and winter in the United States; also *saumya.*

Vishama Agni: The pathologically variable state of the digestive fire or *Agni.*

Vishaya-Shakti: The intrinsic power of *Manas* that impels ordinary attention toward an alluring attraction to the world of sensory objects; the hypnotic pull and glamour of the material world.

Vishesha: Opposites balance each other; one of the two fundamental principles of Ayurvedic treatment; specific.

Vishnu: Deity mentioned in the *Rig-Veda;* later, viewed as the second of the three major Hindu deities (Brahma, Vishnu, Shiva) and considered the sustainer of the universe.

Vishuddha Chakra: The energy node located in the region of the throat.

Vitiation: Impairment, disturbance, or excitation of a *dosha* that may act as a factor leading to the development of disease.

Vivarana: Rapid pervasive and dispersive action.

Viveka: The capacity to properly discriminate that which is real and enduring from the illusory, superficial, and transient phenomena of experience.

Vriddha: Older age.

Vritti: The unstable and irregular oscillations of thoughts within mental processes; a negative connotation describing the untamed mind.

Vyabhichari: Very mild stimuli that may cause disease.

Vyadhikshamatva: Immunity.

Vyakti: The stage of manifestation of a disease.

Vyana Vata: The subdosha of Vata that propels bodily materials in an outward direction; the subdosha that energizes circulation and outward movements.

Yajamana: The one who offers a ritual sacrifice.

Yajna: Sacrificial offering.

Yajur-Veda: One of the four primary Vedas (c. 1,000 B.C.) that contains sacrificial formulas to be chanted during the performance of sacred rituals.

Yajus: Ritual prayers and formulas, especially those derived from the *Rig-Veda*.

Yama: The self-discipline, especially in regard to others, achieved through the practice of the five behavioral guidelines enumerated in the first level of Yoga practice known by the same name.

Yang: A fundamental concept in Chinese medicine connoting the principles of outward movement, solidity, heat, and masculine qualities.

Yappa: Diseases that are chronic but manageable over time.

Yin: A fundamental concept in Chinese medicine connoting the principles of inward movement, fluidity, coolness, and female qualities.

Yoga: In Sanskrit means yoke or union; one of the six major, orthodox Hindu *darshanas;* a system of practice in which an individual strives, through strict self-discipline, to achieve ever greater degrees of connectedness or harnessing to God; the major system of Hindu self-development formulated in the *Yoga Sutras* of Patanjali.

Yoga Sutras: The collection of *sutras* (c. second century B.C. to fourth century A.D.) associated with the name of Patanjali that delineate the classical Yoga system.

Yogatattva: Famous Yoga Upanishad (c. 100 B.C.-A.D. 300) that describes the earliest known forms of varied, pre-classical Yoga practices.

Yukti: The creation of a substance, process, or effect resulting from the confluence of a wide variety of etiological factors; i.e., materials, place, timing, etc.

REFERENCES

Acharya, N. R., & Pandurang, S. (Eds.). (1945). *Sushruta Samhita*. Bombay: Nirnaya Sagar Press.

Anandamurti, S. S. (1993). *Discourses on Tantra* (Vol. 1). Bombay: Ananda Marga Publications.

Anandamurti, S. S. (1994). *Discourses on Tantra* (Vol. 2). Bombay: Ananda Marga Publications.

Apte, V. S. (1993). *The student's Sanskrit-English dictionary*. Delhi: Motilal Banarsidass. (Original work published 1970)

Aurobindo, S. (1976). *The synthesis of Yoga*. Pondicherry, India: Sri Aurobindo Ashram.

Bedekar, V. M., & Palsule, G. B. (Eds.). (1995). *Sixty Upanishads of the Veda*. Delhi: Motilal Banarsidass.

Bender, E. (1967). *Hindi grammar and reader*. Philadelphia: University of Pennsylvania Press.

Bhishagratna, K. L. (Trans.). (1968). *Sushruta Samhita*. Varanasi, India: Chowkhamba Sanskrit Series.

Biardeau, M. (Ed.). (1989). *Hinduism, the anthropology of a civilization*. New Delhi: Oxford University Press.

Block, N., Flanagan, O., & Guzeldere, G. (1997). *The nature of consciousness*. Boston, MA: MIT Press.

Bloomfield, M. (1967). *Hymns of the Athara Veda, SBE 42*. Delhi: MLBD. (Original work published 1897)

Buitenen, J. A. B. (Trans.). (1973–1978). *The Mahabharata* (Vols. 1–3). Chicago and London: University of Chicago Press.

Buitenen, J. A. B. (1981). *The Bhagavadgita in the Mahabharata*. Chicago and London: University of Chicago Press.

Cairns-Smith, A. G. G. (1996). *Evolving the mind: On the nature of matter and the origin of consciousness*. Cambridge: Cambridge University Press.

Chen, K. (1984). *Buddhism in China*. Princeton, NJ: Princeton University Press.

Clifford, T. (1984). *Tibetan Buddhist medicine and psychiatry*. York Beach, ME: Samuel Weiser.

Condron, D. R. (1991). *Dreams of the soul: The Yogi Sutras of Patanjali*. Windyville, MI: SOM Publishing.

Corcos, A. F. (1984). Reproduction and heredity beliefs of the Hindus based on their sacred books. *Journal of Heredity, 75* (2), 152–154.

Coward, H. G., & Raja, K. K. (1990). *The philosophy of the Grammarians, Encyclopedia of Indian Philosophies* (Vol. 5). Princeton, NJ: Princeton University Press.

Dales, G., & Kenoyer, J. M. (1993). *Excavations at Mohenjo Daro, Pakistan*. Philadelphia: University of Pennsylvania Museum Monograph.

Das, S. (1984). Sushruta of India: Pioneer in vesicolithotomy. *Urology, 23* (3), 317–319.

Dasgupta, S. (1975). *A history of Indian philosophy* (Vols. 1–5). Delhi: Motilal Banarsidass.

Dasgupta, S. (1989). *A study of Patanjali*. Delhi: Motilal Banarsidass.

Douillard, J. (2000). *The 3/season diet: Solving the mysteries of food cravings, weight loss, and exercise*. New York: Random House.

Dube, K. C. (1979). Nosology and therapy of mental illness in Ayurveda. *Comparative Medicine East West, 6* (3), 208–209.

Dumont, L. (1980). *Homo Hierarchicus: The caste system and its implications*. Chicago and London: University of Chicago Press.

Dwight, W. (1984). *Athara Veda Samhita*. Delhi: Motilal Banarsidass.

Edney, M. H. (1997). *Mapping an empire: The geographical construction of British India, 1765–1843*. Chicago & London: University of Chicago Press.

Eliade, M. (1973). *Yoga: Immortality and freedom*. Princeton, NJ: Princeton University Press.

Eliade, M. (1978). *History of religious ideas: Vol. 1. From the Stone Age to the Eleusinian Mysteries*. Chicago & London: University of Chicago Press.

Eliade, M. (1982). *History of religious ideas: Vol. 2. From Gautauma Buddha to the triumph of Christianity*. Chicago & London: University of Chicago Press.

Fairservis, W. A. (1975). *The roots of ancient India*. Chicago & London: University of Chicago Press.

Feuerstein, G. (1989). *The Yoga-Sutra of Patanjali: A new translation and commentary*. Rochester, VT: Inner Traditions International.

Feuerstein, G. (1998). *The Yoga tradition: Its history, literature, philosophy, and practice*. Prescott, AZ: Hohm Press.

Fischer-Schreiber, I., Ehrhard, F. K., & Friedrichs, K. (1994). *The encyclopedia of Eastern philosophy and religion*. Boston: Shambhala.

Forte, A. O. (1990). *The self and its states: A state of consciousness doctrine in Advaita Vedanta*. Delhi: Motilal Banarsidass.

Frawley, D., & Lad, V. (1986). *The Yoga of herbs*. Twin Lakes, WI: Lotus Press.

Ganapati, S. V. (1992). *Samaveda*. Delhi: Motilal Banarsidass. (Original work published 1982)

Garfield, J. (1995). *The fundamental wisdom of the middle way: Nagarjuna's Mulamadhyamakakarika*. New York & Oxford: Oxford University Press.

Griffith, R. T. H. (1973). *The Rig-Veda*. Delhi: Motilal Banarsidass. (Original work published 1896)

Grossman, J. (1994). The evolution of inhaler technology. *Journal of Asthma, 31* (1), 55–64.

Gurdjieff, G. I. (1963). *Meetings with remarkable men*. London: Routledge & Kegan Paul.

Hajicek-Dobberstein, S. (1995). Soma siddhas and alchemical enlightment: Psychedelic mushrooms in Buddhist tradition. *Journal of Ethnopharmacology, 48* (2), 99–118.

Haldipur, C. V. (1984). Madness in ancient India: Concept of insanity in Charaka Samhita (1st century A.D.). *Comprehensive Psychiatry, 25* (3), 335–344.

Haldipur, C. V. (1989). Psychiatric nosology and taxonomy in ancient India. *Acta Psychiatrica Scandinavia, 80* (2), 148–150.

Hameroff, S. R., Kaszniak, A. W., & Scott, A. C. (Eds.). (1996). *Toward a science of consciousness*. Boston, MA: MIT Press.

Harishastri, B. (Ed.). (1939). *Vagbhata- Ashtanga Hridaya*. Bombay: Nirnaya Sagar Press.

Hauben, D. J., Baruchin, A., & Mahler, A. (1982). On the history of the free skin graft. *Annals of Plastic Surgery, 9* (3), 242–245.

Heesterman, J. C. (1993). *The broken world of sacrifice: Essays in ancient Indian ritual*. Chicago & London: University of Chicago Press.

Hiltebeitel, A. (1999). *Rethinking India's oral and classical epics*. Chicago & London: University of Chicago Press.

Jamison, S. W. (1991). *Ravenous hyenas and the wounded sun: Myth and ritual in ancient India*. Ithaca, NY: Cornell University Press.

Jee, H. H. Bhagvat Sinh (1993). *Aryan medical science*. New Delhi: D.K. Publishers. (Original work published 1895)

Jha, G. (Trans.). (1984). *The Nyaya-Sutras of Gautama*. Delhi: Motilal Banarsidass.

Johnson, W. (1994). *The Bhagavadgita*. Oxford: Oxford University Press.

Joshi, S. V. (1996). *Ayurveda and Pancharkarma.* Twin Lakes, WI: Lotus Press.

Kadar, S. (1996). *The colors of violence: Cultural identities, religion, and conflict.* Chicago & London: University of Chicago Press.

Kaelber, W. O. (1989). *Tapta Marga: Asceticism and initiation in Vedic India.* Albany, NY: State University of New York Press.

Kak, S. (1987). On the chronology of ancient India. *Indian Journal of the History of Science, 22* (3), 51–62.

Kalupahana, D. J. (1986). *Nagarjuna: The philosophy of the middle way.* Albany, NY: State University of New York Press.

Kansupada, K. B., & Sassani, J. W. (1997). Sushruta: The father of Indian surgery and ophthalmology. *Doctoral Ophthalmology, 93* (1–2), 159–167.

Kaviratna, A. C. (1902–1925). *Charaka Samhita* (Vols. 1–4). Calcutta: Girish Chandra Chakravarti Deva Press.

Kripal, J. (1998). *Kali's child: The mystical and the erotic in the life and teachings of Ramakrishna.* Chicago & London: University of Chicago Press.

Lad, V. (1984). *Ayurveda: The science of self-healing.* Twin Lakes, WI: Lotus Press.

Lad, V. (1996). *Secrets of the pulse: The ancient art of Ayurvedic pulse diagnosis.* Albuquerque, NM: Ayurvedic Press.

Lamm, N. (1986). *Faith and doubt: Studies in traditional Jewish thought.* New York: Ktav Publishing House.

Lele, R. D. (1986). *Ayurveda and modern medicine.* Bombay: Bharratiya Vidya Bhavan.

Lele, A., Ranade, S., & Qutab, A. (1997). *Pancha-Karma and Ayurvedic massage.* Pune: International Academy of Ayurveda.

Lindtner, C. (1997). *Master of wisdom: Writings of the Buddhist Master Nagarjuna.* Berkeley, CA: Dharma Publishing.

Lipner, J. (1994). *Hindus: Their religious beliefs and practices.* London: Routledge.

Mahdihassan, S. (1981). The tradition of alchemy in India. *American Journal of Chinese Medicine, 9* (1), 23–33.

Mahdihassan, S. (1985a). Cinnabar-gold as the best alchemical drug of longevity, called Makaradhwaja in India. *American Journal of Chinese Medicine, 13* (1–4), 93–108.

Mahdihassan, S. (1985b). Indian and Chinese cosmologies reconsidered. *American Journal of Chinese Medicine, 13* (1–4), 5–12.

Mahdihassan, S. (1989). The five cosmic elements as depicted in Indian and Chinese cosmologies. *American Journal of Chinese Medicine, 17* (3–4), 245–252.

Manyam, B. V. (1990). Paralysis agitans and levodopa in "Ayurveda": Ancient Indian medical treatise. *Movement Disorders, 5* (1), 47–48.

Mead, G. R. S. (1895). *Selected works of Plotinus.* London: G. Bell & Sons.

Mead, G. R. S. (1913). *Quests old and new.* London: G. Bell & Sons.

Mehta, P. M. (Ed.). (1949). *Charaka Samhita.* Jamnagar, Gujarat: Gulab Kunverba Society.

Miller, L., & Miller, B. (1995). *Ayurveda and aromatherapy.* Twin Lakes, WI: Lotus Press.

Mishra, R. S. (1959). *Fundamentals of Yoga.* New York: Julian Press.

Mishra, R. S. (1963). *The textbook of Yoga psychology.* New York: Julian Press.

Moos, Vayaskara N. S. (Ed. & Trans.). (1984). *Vagbhata's Ashtanga Hridaya Samhita.* Kerala: Vaidyasarathy Press.

Morningstar, A., & Desai, U. (1990). *The Ayurvedic cookbook.* Twin Lakes, WI: Lotus Press.

Mukerjee, A. B. (1974). The concept of nutrition—Ancient and modern. *Journal of Indian Medical Association, 62* (7), 250–251.

Muller, M. (1899). *The six systems of Indian philosophy.* London: Longmans, Green.

Murthy, K. R. Srikanta (Trans.). (1987). *Madhava Nidanam.* Varanasi: Chaukhambha.

Narang, S. (1984). *The Vaisnava philosophy.* Delhi: Nag Publishers.

Narasimhan, C. V. (Ed.). (1997). *The Mahabharata.* New York: Columbia University Press.

Neumann, E. (1954). *The origins and history of consciousness.* Princeton, NJ: Princeton University Press.

Nichter, L. S., Morgan, R. F., & Nichter, M. A. (1983). The impact of Indian methods for total nasal reconstruction. *Clinical Plastic Surgery, 10* (4), 635–647.

Ninivaggi, F. J. (1999). Attention / Deficit-Hyperactivity Disorder in children and adolescents: Rethinking diagnosis and treatment implications for complicated cases. *Connecticut Medicine, 63* (9), 515–521.

Oberoi, H. (1995). *The construction of religious boundaries.* Chicago & London: University of Chicago Press.

O'Flaherty, W. D. (1981). *The Rig Veda: An anthology.* London: Penguin Books.

Olivelle, P. (1992). *The Samnyasa Upanishads, Hindu scriptures on asceticism and renunciation.* New York & Oxford: Oxford University Press.

Osho, R. (1994). *Heartbeat of the absolute: Discourses on the Ishavasya Upanishad.* Boston, MA: Element.

Osho, R. (1995). *Returning to the source: Talks on Zen*. Boston, MA: Element.

Osho, R. (1996). *Meditation: The first and last freedom: A practical guide to meditation*. New York: St. Martin's Press.

Parpola, A. (1994). *Deciphering the Indus script*. Cambridge, U.K.: Cambridge University Press.

Porter, R. (1997). *The greatest benefit to mankind: The history of medicine*. New York: W. W. Norton.

Potter, K. H. (Ed.). (1994). *Indian philosophical analysis: Nyaya-Vaisesika from Gangesa to Raghunatha Siromani: Vol. 6. Encyclopedia of Indian philosophies*. Princeton, NJ: Princeton University Press.

Prabhupada, Swami (A. C. Bhaktivedanta). (1997). *Bhagavad-Gita as it is*. New York & Los Angeles: Baktivedanta Book Trust.

Prakash, U. B. (1978). Sushruta of ancient India. *Surgical Gynecology & Obstetrics, 146* (2), 263–272.

Radhakrishnan, S. (Trans.). (1953). *The principal Upanishads*. London: Unwin Hyman.

Ranade, S. (1993). *Natural healing through Ayurveda*. Salt Lake City, Utah: Passage Press.

Ranade, S., Ranade, S., Qutab, A., & Deshpande, R. (1997). *Health and disease in Ayurveda and Yoga*. Pune: Anmol Prakashan.

Ray, P., & Gupta, H. N. (1965). *Charaka Samhita: A scientific synopsis*. New Delhi: National Institute of Sciences of India.

Sarkar, S. P. R. (1993). *Yogic treatments and natural remedies*. Calcutta: Ananda Marga Publications.

Savithri, S. R. (1987). Speech pathology in ancient India—A review of Sanskrit literature. *Journal of Communication Disorders, 20* (6), 437–445.

Sharma, P. V. (1976). *Introduction to Dravyaguna*. Varanasi: Chaukhambha Orientalia.

Sharma, P. V. (1977). *Yogaratnamala of Nagarguna*. Varansi: Chaukhambha Orientalia.

Sharma, P. V. (1995). *Caraka-Samhita* (Vols. 1–4). Varanasi: Chaukhambha Orientalia.

Sigerist, H. E. (1951). *A history of medicine: Vol. 1. Primitive and archaic medicine*. New York: Oxford University Press.

Sigerist, H. E. (1961). *A history of medicine: Vol. 2. Early Greek, Hindu, and Persian medicine*. New York: Oxford University Press.

Singer, C., & Underwood, E. A. (1962). *A short history of medicine* (2nd ed.). New York: Oxford University Press.

Sivaraman, K. (1973). *Saivism in philosophical perspective: A study of the formative concepts, problems and methods of Saiva Siddhanta*. Delhi: Motilal Banarsidass.

Solso, R. L. (1999). *Mind and brain sciences in the 21st century*. Boston, MA: MIT Press.

Staal, F. (1963). Sanskrit and Sanskritization. *Journal of Asian Studies, 23* (3), 261–275.

Staal, F. (1983). *Agni. The Vedic ritual of the Fire Altar* (Vols. 1–2). Berkeley: University of California Press.

Staal, F. (1989). *Rules without meaning, ritual, mantras and the human sciences*. New York: Peter Lang.

Steiner, R. (1964). *The philosophy of freedom*. New York: Anthroposophic Press. (Original work published 1884)

Steiner, R. (1968). *A theory of knowledge*. New York: Anthroposophic Press. (Original work published 1886)

Svoboda, R. E. (1989). *Prakruti: Your Ayurvedic constitution*. Albuquerque, NM: Geocom.

Svoboda, R. E. (1992). *Ayurveda: Life, health and longevity*. London: Arkana Penguin Books.

Trikamji, J., & Ram, N. (1980). *Sushruta Samhita of Sushruta*. Varanasi: Chaukhambha Orientalia.

Unschuld, P. U. (1979). The Chinese reception of Indian medicine in the first millennium A.D. *Bulletin of the History of Medicine, 53* (3), 329–345.

Unschuld, P. U. (1985). *Medicine in China*. Berkeley: University of California Press.

Urbach, E. E. (1979). *The sages: Their concepts and beliefs*. Cambridge, MA: Harvard University Press.

Vesci, U. (1992). *Heat and sacrifice in the Vedas*. Delhi: Motilal Banarsidass.

Vishnudevananda, S. (1960). *The complete illustrated book of Yoga*. New York: Julian Press.

White, D. G. (1996). *The alchemical body: Siddha traditions in medieval India*. Chicago & London: University of Chicago Press.

Whitney, W. D., & Lanman, C. R. (1996). *Athara Veda Samhita: Translation with critical and exegetical commentary*. Delhi: Motilal Banarsidass. (Original work published 1905)

Williams, P. (1989). *Mahayana Buddhism: The doctrinal foundations*. London & New York: Routledge.

Wiseman, N., & Ellis, A. (1985). *Fundamentals of Chinese medicine*. Brookline, MA: Paradigm Publications.

Wohlberg, J. (1990). Haoma-Soma in the world of ancient Greece. *Journal of Psychoactive Drugs, 22* (3), 333–342.

Yogananda, P. (1946). *Autobiography of a Yogi*. Los Angeles, CA: Self Realization Fellowship.

Yukteswar, S. (1990). *The holy science*. Los Angeles: Self-Realization Fellowship. (Original work published 1894)

Zaehner, R. C. (1961). *Mysticism sacred and profane*. New York: Oxford University Press.

Zaehner, R. C. (1966). *Hinduism*. New York: Oxford University Press.

Zimmer, H. (1951). *Philosophies of India*. Princeton, NJ: Princeton University Press.